**THE
ROAD BACK
PROGRAM**

HOW TO GET OFF
CYMBALTA® SAFELY

There is Hope. There is a Solution...

JAMES HARPER

How to Get Off Cymbalta Safely

Copyright 2005 - TX-6-486-774, 2006, TX-6-607-303, 2007, 2009

All rights reserved. No part of this book may be reproduced or transmitted in any form or by any means without written permission of the author.

ISBN 1441484426

DEDICATION

To my mother, I thank you from the bottom of my heart. As a child you gave me a safe space to just be a child and allowed me to stumble and learn from my mistakes. As an adult you encouraged me to keep looking for new answers. With your passing this past year you have helped me learn value in each moment. Thank you and you are missed.

To my love, best friend and wife. This book would never have been written without you. This program would never have been developed without you. Your insistence in the early days is why The Road Back Program is here. Thank you.

To those of you that are about to use the material in this book to overcome Cymbalta adverse reactions. May your journey be one of comfort and positive change. You can make it.

DISCLAIMER

The claims, information and products mentioned in this book, *How to Get Off Cymbalta Safely,* have not been evaluated by the United States Food and Drug Administration and are not approved to diagnose, treat, cure or prevent disease.

The information provided in the book, *How to Get Off Cymbalta Safely*, is for informational purposes only and is not intended as a substitute for advice from your physician or other healthcare professional.

You should not use the information in this book for diagnosis or treatment of any health problem or for prescription of any medication or other treatment.

You should consult with a healthcare professional before starting any diet, exercise or supplementation program, before taking any medication, or if you have, or suspect that you might have a health problem.

A NOTE FROM THE AUTHOR

Since 1999 when The Road Back Program, How to Get Off Psychiatric Drugs Safely, was released to the general public, tens of thousands of people have successfully tapered off their psychiatric medications using The Road Back Program.

You may have been prescribed Cymbalta for a non-mental health reason; however, Cymbalta is a psychoactive medication and must be treated as such.

This book is written for individuals, pharmacists and healthcare providers, *How to Get Off Cymbalta Safely* is specific to Cymbalta. Thousands of people around the world are using this information every day in their battle to successfully free themselves of debilitating Cymbalta side effects.

I want to acknowledge the many of people, from the four corners of Earth and all walks of life, who have successfully come off Cymbalta using this program. Their perseverance and feedback have helped advance this program to today's high degree of success.

And I applaud you, opening this book for the first time, for your courage and resolve to change your life and get yourself back as your reward.

I understand the apprehension you may feel about deciding to come off Cymbalta, especially if you have tried to do so before and failed, or if you have heard horror stories of others who have tried to come off Cymbalta.

Further, I understand the questions you might be asking at this point:

- *Will I experience mental or physical pain while on this program?*
- *Will I have other side effects while on this program?*
- *Will the Cymbalta side effects get worse before they get better?*

- *Will my depression get worse during this program?*
- *Will my anxiety levels increase?*

You may have many other questions in addition to those above, but most importantly you should know that I have formulated The Road Back Program to be virtually side effect free. The testament to this, as you will see throughout the book, is that people just like you start to feel better, both mentally and physically, from day one.

The Road Back Program is set-up so that you only start reducing the Cymbalta after you feel a major positive change and all or nearly all-existing side effects from the Cymbalta are eliminated. Thus, you know from the very beginning change is possible, that this time there is a chance for you, and that you *can* do this and feel well once again. That's why I have called it "The Road Back" – it is a route that will take you back where you want to be.

The Road Back Program is simple, effective, and extremely powerful: when applied correctly. You too can have resounding success in getting off Cymbalta and getting your life back.

Based on extensive research, specific "super foods" have been formulated for this program. Their use, in conjunction with the full and complete Road Back Program, have resulted in an estimated 80% success rate of people getting off their psychiatric medications, while also enormously reducing the potential and feared side effects from withdrawal.

What unwanted feelings come from you and what feelings does Cymbalta generate? The Road Back Program separates these confusing symptoms, and once this separation occurs, the real you emerges.

One major change most people experience with The Road Back; their reach for life returns or truly begins for the first time. Reach is defined as: to extend out; to touch or to seize; to communicate with.

Life is defined as: the quality that distinguishes a *vital* and functional being from a dead body or inanimate matter (Webster's Dictionary). Per the definition of life, *you* are vital. We need you and humankind needs you. The positive changes you can bring to others are beyond imagining. Life can be grand, life can be fulfilling; you, changing your life and having "reach" return will absolutely affect others in your environment.

Reach can return with your children, spouse, work or activities you have been putting off for years that you have always wanted to do, or to do once again.

Remember and hold the following close to your heart as you travel The Road Back:

- You Can Change.
- You Can Change How You Feel.
- You Can Be a Positive Influence for Others.
- You Can Make It.

As you read this book, perhaps you might be thinking "...this sounds good for others..." or "...others can make it, but not me..." Believe me, I am referring directly to you.

My best to you in your journey,

Jim Harper
Founder
The Road Back

CONTENTS

1. The Road Back Basics 1
2. The Four Simple Steps 5
3. "Super Foods" Used on The Road Back Program 7
4. Cymbalta Side Effects Defined………………………………...22
5. Things to Be Aware of... 47
6. General Pre-Tapering and Tapering Instructions 51
7. Daily Journal 67
8. Graph Your Success.. 71
9. Pre-Taper for Benzodiazepines, Anti-anxiety, Anticonvulsants and Sleep Medication 73
10. Pre-Taper for Cymbalta 93
11. How to Taper Off Benzodiazepines, Anti-anxiety, Anticonvulsants and Sleep Medications *(Slow and Gradual Taper)* 119
12. How to Taper Off Benzodiazepines, Anti-anxiety, Anticonvulsants and Sleep Medications *(Fast and Gradual Taper)* 127
13. How to Taper Off Cymbalta *(Slow and Gradual Taper)* .. 139
14. How to Taper Off Cymbalta *(Fast and Gradual Taper)* ... 147
15. Once Off Cymbalta 147
16. Already Started to Taper Cymbalta or Quit Cold Turkey 155
17. How to Taper Off Multiple Medications 159
18. What Can Be Done if You Have Never Taken Psychiatric Medication 165

19. The Science Behind The Road Back 169

Glossary 191
References 225
Flow Charts 241
    Pre-Taper Flow Chart if You Have Daytime Anxiety,
    Agitation or Insomnia 243
    Pre-Taper if You Have Fatigue and
    Do Not Have Anxiety or Insomnia 253
    Pre-Taper Benzodiazepines, Anti-Anxiety,
    Anticonvulsant and Sleep Medication 259

CHAPTER 1

THE ROAD BACK BASICS

"When I first read your website, I thought no way. This is too simple. Barley? Give me a break. I figured I really didn't have anything to lose. I felt like crap warmed over anyway. Two weeks later and I mean two weeks later, I am a new man! The fog has cleared, the depression is gone, and my wife has a husband again. Barley, who would have thought? Needless to say, I was not surprised when the Omega 3 and Body Calm did exactly what you said they would. Thank you from the bottom of my big Texas heart."

T.D.
Austin, TX.

People from all over the world send in testimonials like this every day, praising The Road Back Program and how it has helped them regain their hold on life. Often, as this man said, the program at first seems too simple. When something is simple, there could be a tendency to disbelieve results. Nevertheless, the Road Back Program IS simple, while also highly effective when followed using the correct supplements, and completing all steps.

The Road Back Program is a very specific, heavily researched, proven program. As noted above, I formulated this program to help people get off all kinds of drugs, while reducing to almost zero the crippling side effects often associated with coming off the drugs.

Newly formulated psychiatric medications seem to incessantly roll out of research labs into distribution. But I have found over the years that no matter what the drug's formulation, The Road Back Program is still effective. Since you are reading this book you most likely understand, firsthand, the devastating side effects of Cymbalta. As of today, tens of thousands of people over the world have used The Road Back Program to free themselves from those crippling bonds.

Which Side Effects Are You Suffering From?

Due to the widely varying circumstances of the many people who will read this book, I have outlined several scenarios delineating where you might now stand, and how The Road Back Program will apply to you. Establishing your current particular circumstances will be of great benefit and provide a starting point for your progress on The Road Back Program.

Scenario One:
You are not on any psychiatric medications, and never have been, but are thinking about taking these medications:

Debate and statistics hit the news nearly every day about the effectiveness or potential harm caused by psychiatric drugs. The confusions tend to mount further when the latest clinical trial results counters the evidence published just last month.

I am not about to enter the fray of the psychiatric drug debate with this book. The intent here is to offer hope and solutions for those desiring to safely taper off psychiatric medication as well as offer a few solutions to those seeking an alternative to psychiatric medication.

THE ROAD BACK BASICS

If you are looking for a solution rather than taking a psychiatric drug, this book offers nutritional answers and a simple blood test that may provide the better way you are seeking. That word "may," should be capitalized, italicized, underlined, put in bold type and double-sized.

Certainly, while nutrition is not the answer for all of the ills that might beset our lives, neither is a drug the answer.

If your symptoms are caused or perpetuated by deficiencies in a specific or broad range of vitamins, amino acids, fatty acids, enzymes, protein, etc, then this part of the program will probably be the answer for you.

Scenario Two:
You are taking Cymbalta and want to withdraw from the drug:

You are a prime candidate for The Road Back Program. You may or may not be experiencing side effects from the Cymbalta. You may or may not have tried to taper before. You may have been on Cymbalta for a few days or many years.

You will find tremendous benefit and success with The Road Back Program.

Scenario Three:
You have started to taper off and are suffering:

Dr. Donald E. McAlpine, Psychiatry and Psychology, Mayo Clinic notes: *"It's important to taper off slowly, extending the taper over several weeks under your physician's direction. When you stop too quickly, you may experience so-called discontinuation symptoms, which can masquerade as relapse."*

The Road Back Program has been designed to help you get back on track and succeed with the tapering process. This can take a little more time initially, but there IS a way back.

Scenario Four:
You have already tapered off Cymbalta and are still suffering, or stopped Cymbalta "cold turkey":

Due to the nature and composition of Cymbalta and the effects on the body, withdrawal side effects can plague you long after complete withdrawal. Such "protracted" or continuing withdrawal side effects are probably the most difficult situation to deal with. The Road Back Program can be effective and successful in eliminating these side effects from your life.

Stopping Cymbalta "cold turkey" or tapering off too quickly cause many of the same side effects, and often to the same magnitude. This situation usually requires the longest road back, but can be accomplished. Many people start to feel better one week into the program and reach a major positive change by the fourteenth day of the program.

Scenario Five:
You have all four of the points listed below:

In the past, The Road Back could not help a person who fit the following four points. Today we have a program for you as well.

These four points are:

1. You are sensitive to all supplements and most foods.

2. You came off Cymbalta and suffered *extreme* withdrawal symptoms.

3. You are still experiencing "protracted" withdrawals, even though off Cymbalta.

4. You have been off Cymbalta for at least six months.

Simply follow the pre-taper program for the medication(s) you took.
Once you have reached a point of no side effects remaining, continue with the nutritional supplements for 45 additional days.

I urge you to not give up hope. This program will get you fully recovered from the medication.

CHAPTER 2

THE FOUR SIMPLE STEPS

"My God! I took the Power Barley and the Omega 3 this morning and it is as if thousands of pounds of weight were just lifted from my body. I feel bright, energetic but not hyper. This is truly amazing. I read the testimonials on your website, and thought maybe for other people this works, but I have tried supplements before. Your wording of well-being now makes sense. I can say for the first time ever I know what it feels like to have the feeling of well-being. It is Christmas morning where I am and I can't thank you enough for the unexpected present."

P.M.
Medford, OR.

Step One

Do Not Stop Cymbalta Abruptly
- Do not "self medicate" (adjust the Cymbalta dosage without consulting your prescribing physician).
- Do not think you are somehow "different" regarding Cymbalta and think you can cut the Cymbalta by 50%, drop two meds at one time or skip days of the medication, etc.

- Keep it simple; follow the program.
- If you are doing well and seeing results, do not change anything. Just stay on the program.
- Remember that The Road Back Program is a systematic process.

Step Two

Find Out What You Will Need for the Program

- Go to Chapter Three or *www.theroadback.org,* which lists all the supplements that you will need for this Cymbalta program.

Print off this list or write it down and review the ingredients contained in the "super foods" you will be taking.

Step Three

Get a Complete Physical

- Schedule a complete physical with your doctor.
- Take this book with you and review the program with your doctor.
- Have your physician rule out any physical illness or disease.

Step Four

Purchase Your Super Food Supplements and Get Started

- Call TRB Health offices 1 + (866) 810-3809, or *www.trbhealth.com,* and purchase the products needed for your program. Check with TRB Health for a healthcare provider or store near you that carries all products needed for the full taper program.
- Start taking your supplements as outlined in the guidelines that pertain to your personal scenario.

CHAPTER 3

"SUPER FOODS" USED ON THE ROAD BACK PROGRAM

"I am now more than halfway off my antidepressant, using the program. I was able to reduce a little bit of the medication with my naturopath, but we reached a standstill after the second reduction. The side effects started and we could not get rid of them. The Omega 3 got rid of the brain zaps within a few hours and they never came back. The Body Calm has been amazing at helping me stay calm during the day and with my sleep. And that barley did just what you said it would do for my energy and complete feelings. I can't thank you enough."

J.S.
New York

The Basic Nutritional Premise

The body is an amazing and complex instrument, designed to deal with the rigors of life, as long as it is cared for properly. However, when the body's chemistry or systems are altered, the body will fight back to balance out the attack.

Supply your body with the foods necessary to sustain health and life, give your body foods dense in nutritional value, address the body as a whole, rather than as a piecemeal project, and you will benefit from and feel the marvelous results of your attentions.

One of the reasons why The Road Back Program suggests only the nutritional products listed in this chapter is that just any supplement off the shelf may not be nutrient filled and thus not easily assimilate, worsening your chance of great results.

Over more than a decade I have spent thousands of hours researching the correct and most basic nutrient system for The Road Back Program. From this research, I concluded that not just food, but "super foods" are required during the tapering process off psychiatric medications. "Super foods" are highly nutritious supplements considered to contain the complete array of all vitamins, minerals, and amino acids a human body needs.

How The Program Works

Your body naturally triggers a self-protective inflammatory process. This natural function responds to normal activities such as exercise, fighting off toxins, allergies, illness, incorrect foods, weight gain, medications - you name it.

For example, a sore throat or infected cut. The area becomes red and inflamed as the body rushes microscopic "fire fighters" to the area to contain and put out the fire and to then start the healing process.

But if your body gets overloaded and can no longer control the inflammation, or more basically lacks enough "fire fighters" to douse the flames, then an internal switch flips, and your systems can start going awry, ultimately resulting in an overall imbalance.

If you have a physical condition, including menopause, weight gain, diabetes or so many others, and then throw Cymbalta on top, you can be adding fuel to an already burning fire. In essence, you flip the switch that overloads your body so it can no longer function as intended.

Starting from this premise, I ventured out on my nutritional quest, looking for a nutritional undercut, to find the most basic and simple physical and nutritional needs. My goal? To calm down the systems of the body naturally, while stopping the inflammation; to stop the suffering caused by the very medications that might be causing, or contributing to, the problems.

After these nutrients are introduced into the body, the internal fire dies down, the body re-gains control, and the healing process starts from within. This premise led to the discovery and development of the "super foods" now comprising The Road Back Program.

While my nutritional research continues, the "super foods" now formulated for The Road Back Program provide the most nutritionally complete cellular support currently available, allowing for the most complete assimilation and absorption. These "super foods" undercut genetic makeup, providing most people, whether on Cymbalta or not, vast benefit.

As a note, your genetic makeup is a unique microscopic combination of DNA, which are chemical compounds determining the unique physical traits of each living thing.

The area of nutrition can be littered with confusing words and information so technical, it can seem overwhelming. I have tried to simplify and distill what you need to know, so you can proceed with The Road Back Program understanding the basic premise and how "super foods" work in your body to counteract the drugs' damage.

Thousands of people worldwide have stood where you now stand; ready to take their lives back and free themselves from Cymbalta and the resulting side effects. While every person is unique and life offers no guarantees, if you follow this program precisely, you should begin to feel better and do better soon after you start.

The following information will ensure the "super foods" taken during your tapering phase provide the most benefit possible.

If you require additional technical information, please read the chapter, The Science Behind The Road Back.

"Super Food" Specifics

> *"I started your program two weeks ago and what a difference! I didn't think you were telling the truth about the products, but I feel like a new woman. Can I stay on the products for life after the taper is over? Thank you for your efforts. You all are a godsend"*
>
> *L.V.*
> *Reno, Nevada*

These foods are so effective because they are simple, pure, strong and bursting with whole-food nutrition. To quote "super food" guru David Sandoval, "You may exercise your body, but super foods exercise your cells."

When I started my research into the psychiatric drug tapering problem, I relied on available, over-the-counter nutritional products to help people with their tapering programs. As with any other research, there were ups and downs to this approach, because I learned that over-the-counter nutritional products were often either too harsh, or just not of the quality needed to accomplish the task. I soon realized that I needed to formulate the specific combinations required, and must find a company with the highest standards available to manufacture these nutritional products exactly as specified.

The products recommended for The Road Back Program are produced by TRB Health and a few select additional manufacturers. These products include, among others are Power Barley Formula, Ultimate Omega 3, Body Calm capsules (or liquid), Essential Protein Formula, RenewPro, Probiotic Supreme, Calsorption, Nature's Vitamin C, CalesiumD and Vitamin E. If you have ever taken a barley product, Omega 3, or protein drink before and then try the TRB Health products, you typically will notice the positive difference within a day.

An enormous number of supplements, vitamins, and other beneficial health-related products are available today. A list so long that it can seem impossible to decide what to purchase. But for the success of The Road

Back Program, I have sidestepped that list, as they did not meet my criteria: success in helping people taper off their psychiatric medications, one for one, each and every time.

What I found is that throwing random, unrelated health products into your body during any form of withdrawal from Cymbalta, would create at best, a "willy-nilly," disordered, unpredictable response, or in the worst case scenario extreme illness. While some *might* benefit from such an approach, the vast majority will not achieve the desired results, even worse could create new problems for themselves and their loved ones in the process.

My goal is to help you safely taper off Cymbalta, while dramatically reducing the side effects of your medication, as well as the side effects of withdrawal.

What works are the correct "super foods," introduced into your body in the correct amounts at the correct times throughout the day, so the side effects of the Cymbalta and the tapering process are minimized, while concurrently the relief is increased.

Specific "super foods," taken in an exact order at specific times will counter-balance and eliminate side effects. The path that stops those side effects is The Road Back Program.

One very common side effect created by Cymbalta is extreme body aches and pains as well as intestinal upset. These supplements are designed to ease the suffering caused by Cymbalta and they will address these side effects as well. Do not underestimate the impact the Probiotic Supreme can have. The intestinal tract is where all nutrients must first pass before absorption and an intestinal tract malfunction of any type will create havoc through the entire body, not just in the gut area.

Beta 1, 3-D Glucan

Beta 1, 3-D Glucan is part of the tapering program if you have anxiety, insomnia but not depression. If you are taking Cymbalta for depression you should not use the Beta 1, 3-D Glucan.

The human immune system includes a substance called IL-2. Individuals with low levels of IL-2 will have anxiety and problems with sleep. Stage 2 of sleep requires a sufficient level of IL-2 for a deep restful sleep.

Beta 1, 3-D Glucan has been clinically proven to not only increase levels of IL-2 in the human immune system but to keep the IL-2 levels increased for an extended time after the product is discontinued.

Body Calm

One of the most common complaints of people either on Cymbalta or those who are trying to come off Cymbalta is daytime anxiety and inability to achieve normal sleep at night. Sleep is an integral part of life, helps to stabilize mood, foster clear thinking and assist with reaction time. Sleep gives the body a chance to rebuild. Even though your body is doing a lot of work while you sleep, you should not be. Without plenty of restful sleep, daily functioning can be miserable.

Now, take your situation. Your body is already stressed from its private war against the Cymbalta being ingested each day. The body is nutritionally stripped of the basic food elements needed for health and proper re-growth of cells, and now you can't sleep. Anyone could understandably be a "basket case" after just a few sleep-deprived nights.

You have hit straight into this catch-22:

The Cymbalta might be creating sleeplessness. Your body's fight to minimize the cause of sleeplessness while the side effects of trying to withdraw also cause sleeplessness.

You cannot win this battle without help. And too often, complaints about sleep are met with a new prescription for yet another side-effect-producing drug. This basic potential psychosis producing problem fueled my hunt for a natural supplement that would promote and easily allow sleep, while at the same time creating no new and unwanted side effects.

I discovered the solution in a product made from tart cherries.

"SUPER FOODS" USED ON THE ROAD BACK PROGRAM

A true miracle food, tart cherries (the proprietary blend of Body Calm) are one of nature's most nutritionally dense, containing a wide variety of powerful anti-oxidants and phyto (plant) chemicals. Tart cherries also have a small amount of naturally occurring melatonin and potassium, both of which are a magic elixir when it comes to addressing anxiety and inability to sleep. Tart cherry products are also highly regarded because their anti-oxidant properties help with inflammation of the joints, aches and pains, cramps, even headaches.

Different from any prescribed medication you may be on or have taken in the past, Body Calm does not knock you out or turn you into a zombie. Taken during the day, Body Calm will help relieve anxiety without making you tired, foggy or having a feeling of not being there. Body Calm taken at night, about an hour before bed, will help you fall asleep naturally. Upon waking in the morning, you won't feel groggy, weary or have to drag yourself out of the sheets. But you *will* feel you've had a restorative, restful sleep.

Body Calm Supreme

Anxiety, stress and insomnia are major Cymbalta withdrawal side effects, comprising the most common side effects for all psychoactive medication, especially during withdrawal. Body Calm Supreme was formulated for use in conjunction with Body Calm to handle anxiety, stress and insomnia. Body Calm Supreme combines 50 mg Body Calm and 200 mg of Passion Flower.

Passion Flower has been shown in several clinical trials during the last decade to handle such things as generalized anxiety, insomnia, and hypertension, withdrawal off benzodiazepines, withdrawal off opiates, narcotics, alcohol and several other addictive substances. Every clinical trial was successful. The same type of Passion Flower used in the clinical trials has been used to formulate Body Calm Supreme. Of course, not all Passion Flower is the same as there are over 500 species of Passion Flower. If you luckily used the correct species, you would still need to pull out of this herb the specific ingredient that achieves these results. The Passion Flower produced by TRB Health is closest to the product used in clinical trials. Nothing else came close.

This discovery and waiting until several of our own test cases could be run delayed the publication of this book by several months. The wait was well worth it. The most difficult cases with anxiety turned around quickly and smoothly; these side effects gone in a few days instead of the usual one or two weeks.

CalesiumD

CalesiumD is a proprietary blend of calcium citrate, magnesium and vitamin D3. The calcium's non-ionic form reduces the chance of calcium induced anxiety or insomnia. Many people taking medication are calcium deficient and have a need for calcium but an ionic form of calcium causes increased anxiety. For the best absorption of calcium, include the Calsorption.

Calsorption

We added Calsorption to our recommended product list for one reason: *calcium absorption*.

Calcium absorption is a major health concern throughout the world. Ads play constantly on television about new food products enriched with calcium. With all that calcium emphasis, why is osteoporosis still on the rise? Why do Americans suffer such with problem when calcium promotes weight loss? Why do so many females suffer debilitating PMS symptoms, pre-menopause, menopause and post-menopause?

Insufficient calcium consumption does not always cause calcium deficiency. Our bodies need to assimilate the calcium taken in and put to use.

At The Road Back, calcium absorption has been on the research agenda for several years. Many people with anxiety that take calcium will have a calcium reaction and instead of the natural calming effect as advertised by most calcium suppliers, these people become overly anxious. Once these people stopped taking calcium, their anxiety level went back down.

But, people taking medication usually need additional calcium because the medication depletes calcium from the body. Many people need to supplement daily with calcium to help with health conditions. They get caught on a "damned if I do and damned if I don't" merry-go-round.

We had to find a way to both improve calcium absorption rates without affecting the metabolism of medication or creating a drug/supplement interaction.

The Road Back found that solution.

What is the Solution?

A food supplement named Calsorption.

What is Calsorption and How Does Calsorption Work?

Calsorption is Inulin, a natural soluble fiber made from chicory roots. Inulin has been shown to increase the quantity of beneficial bacteria in the digestive system. Healthy levels of these important bacteria can result in improved intestinal function, relief of constipation and digestive comfort while also assisting the assimilation of calcium. In addition, Inulin's positive effect on calcium absorption in adolescents and postmenopausal women potentially improves bone health.

Inulin, an all-natural prebiotic, supports optimal colon functioning and mineral absorption. Prebiotics are non-digestible fibers which are the energy source for the beneficial bacteria in the colon. By feeding the beneficial bacteria, we keep our bodies in balance. Inulin, from chicory root, is an easy to disperse fine granulated white powder. Furthermore, with its mildly sweet taste but without surging blood sugar levels, inulin can be used as a sugar replacement in low calorie or diabetic-suitable foods.

What are the health benefits of Calsorption?

Calsorption is a prebiotic fermented in the large intestine by the beneficial bacteria, bifidobacteria. Following the consumption of Inulin, blood sugar levels are not elevated making it a quality sugar substitute in foods for diabetics. Also, as a soluble fiber, Calsorption may help maintain regularity.

What is a prebiotic?

A prebiotic selectively stimulates growth of healthy bacteria in the colon such as Bifidobacteria and Lactobacilli, which provide benefits to the body's digestive system. Inulin is fermented by these intestinal bacteria and short chain fatty acids are produced. *This can then cause a lowering of the pH in the large intestine, and result in increased calcium absorption.* This lower pH also slows the growth of certain bacteria that can weaken the immune system.

How much Calsorption should be consumed each day?

Prebiotic benefits and calcium absorption can be seen from Inulin at 5 grams per day. Add 5 of the 1 gram scoops of Calsorption to water, or any other food or drink, daily for this benefit.

Clinical trials have shown that 5 grams of (Calsorption) Inulin a day will increase the assimilation of calcium by up to 38%. That is a *significant* increase of absorption.

You can find Inulin in several food products. However, 5 grams a day of Inulin are required to cause this positive change with calcium absorption.

There are a few brands now being sold that claim their unique patented product helps with the absorption of calcium. They have simply added a unique substance to Inulin and filed for a patent, but the real benefit is coming from the Inulin. These other added substances are really no more than filler, thus the customer ingests less than 5 grams of Inulin of no true benefit.

"SUPER FOODS" USED ON THE ROAD BACK PROGRAM

The absorption issue with calcium cannot be emphasized enough. Weight loss requires calcium.

CLA *(conjugated linoleic acid)*

CLA is used both as part of our recommended weight loss program and for handling depression and stress. CLA has been clinically shown to significantly lower a specific inflammation marker, IL-6, directly associated with weight loss, depression and Post Traumatic Stress Disorder. CLA has also been shown to reduce the symptom of anxiety.

CLA is Omega 6 oil and must be taken along with an Omega 3 fish oil and vitamin E to maintain the proper balance of Omega 3/6 and for a complete metabolism.

Essential Protein Formula

Protein is a fundamental building block of the body, deriving from both animal and plant sources. Animal sources include fish, chicken, beef as well as dairy products and eggs. Plant sources include beans, soy and soy products, nuts, grains and even some vegetables such as broccoli. However, one of the best sources of protein comes from whey protein isolate, a by-product of turning milk into cheese.

Whey isolate protein has the perfect make up for easy assimilation, resulting in your body getting more of the nutrients in the protein. As well as being an excellent protein source, whey isolate protein acts as an antioxidant, helping support a strong and healthy immune system and balancing out blood sugar levels.

One vicious side effect of Cymbalta - ramping up blood sugar levels while also creating a high-level, internal, acidic environment. Weight gain inevitably results. Stabilized blood sugar levels bring you that much closer to stopping weight gain, then starting weight reduction.

As discussed in the section on Power Barley, the Essential Protein Formula also contains Aktivated Barley, a slow-burning, good carbohydrate that assimilates over approximately four hours. Because of this slow assimilation, blood sugar levels are balanced, preventing energy level "spikes." Instead you will feel sustained energy carrying you through your day.

One of the final ingredients helping the Essential Protein Formula perform its special magic is lecithin, somewhat of a miracle food. Lecithin, among other things, transmits nerve impulses or messages in the brain; helps maintain the structural integrity of the cells, and acts as a natural tranquilizer for glandular exhaustion, as well as nervous and mental disorder. Even more, other benefits include assisting the liver in disposing of the waste filtered through it and helping relieve insomnia. With all these benefits in place, and especially with your blood sugar levels stabilized, you will feel less jittery, experience fewer mood swings and less anxiety. Your brain will calm down as the nerve endings are soothed, making the messages constantly being sent and received more accurate and less chaotic.

Nature's Vitamin C

Today, vitamin C's vital role in everyday health is a given. Questions about what type and how much Vitamin C to take start the viewpoint wars.

Research shows you do not need to take high doses of vitamin C if you take the correct vitamin C and have all the needed amino acids and other vitamins in place. Harvard Medical School ran a clinical trial showing the results from people eating 2 kiwi fruit a day. The vitamin C in kiwi fruit is four times higher than oranges and kiwi-generated vitamin C also assisted with maintaining DNA integrity. Of note, less than 1 kiwi fruit a day was no help and eating more than 2 kiwi fruit a day did not provide additional benefits for the body.

With food sensitivities running out of control and a rather large percentage of the population unable to consume kiwi due to such sensitivities, a different source of natural vitamin C should be used.

For the maximum potential gain from RenewPro (more on this later), a person should have ample amount of vitamin C and vitamin E. The master antioxidant glutathione will freely receive a toxin that has been grabbed by vitamin C and vitamin E and allow the molecule of vitamin C and vitamin E to go back out and grab additional toxins. If the glutathione levels are too low in the body, the vitamin C and vitamin E will hold onto the toxin, not release the toxin, and become toxic themselves.

As long as your cells have glutathione in abundance, only a small amount of the correct vitamin C and E are required.

Vitamin C will help lower inflammation in the body.

If your adrenals are being taxed due to anxiety, stress, depression and fatigue, vitamin C is a must. Vitamin C kick starts the adrenals. Commonly, once the adrenals begin their healing process the feelings of anxiety and stress lessen greatly.

Nature's Vitamin C is the vitamin C to take. An all natural vitamin C and the only vitamin C recommended other than eating 2 kiwi fruit a day.

Power Barley Formula

The Power Barley Formula is comprised of three simple yet powerful ingredients: young green barley, Aktivated Barley™, and carrots all blended into an easily assimilated powdered form. Easy assimilation is key to the nutritional effectiveness of this product, as well as all the other super foods on The Road Back Program.

Power Barley Formula is U.S.D.A. approved. Based on the contents of this formula and an FDA issued statement in December 2005, TRB Health makes the following health claim regarding the Power Barley Formula: "Soluble fiber from foods, such as Power Barley Formula, as part of a diet low in saturated fat and cholesterol, may reduce the risk of heart disease. A serving of Power Barley Formula supplies two grams of the soluble fiber necessary per day to have this effect."

Chlorophyll

Young green barley is a "green food." Its main component – chlorophyll. Chlorophyll, giving plants their green color, is the single most critical substance in plants, allowing light absorption from the sun and conversion into useable energy. This captured energy transfers into higher quality nutrients when ingested, either from fruits and vegetables, or "green foods" such as barley grass juice, wheat grass juice, alfalfa juice, Spirulina, and others. In the Power Barley Formula, chlorophyll neutralizes the high levels of acid that have been created in your body by drugs.

Between a daily diet of highly-processed, high protein/high acid foods and the medications, the acid/alkaline balance in your body has been severely thrown off. When you add young green barley to your diet, the high level of acidity starts to calm down and move back into the balanced range needed to repair damage as well as maintain good health. Green barley gives your body a fighting chance in the tapering process. Other benefits include helping detoxify your liver, while also increasing blood stream oxygen levels.

Famous research scientist, E. Bircher noted, "Chlorophyll is concentrated sun power and it increases the functions of the heart, affects the vascular system, the intestines, the uterus and the lungs. It raises the basic nitrogen exchange and is, therefore, a tonic which, considering its stimulating properties, cannot be compared with any other."

Glutathione and DNA Studies

During my research and DNA studies, I found that roughly 50% of the population has a genetic variation, or inability, to accept and easily use Vitamins B6, B12, and Folate. These vitamins are part of the B complex group, which consists of eight separate B vitamins. While these vitamins can be obtained from separate sources, they are also interdependent on one another. Vitamin B6, Vitamin B12 and Folate (otherwise referred to as folic acid when found in synthetic form) are critical to health and recovery from psychiatric medications because they deal with body systems that have been directly affected by these medications.

Because of this genetic variation, 50 % of the population lacks the components needed to cleanse and detoxify the body, create healthy new cells, and assist with mental and emotional factors. Additionally, the inability to assimilate these vitamins can leave people craving these nutrients. They may try to satisfy this craving by consuming large quantities of foods such as beans, eggs, fish, lentils, meat, soybeans, seeds and yogurt. However, no matter how large the consumption of these foods, the body cannot assimilate all the nutrients, thus is often left still craving the missing nutrients.

B6, B12, and folate also help the body create something called glutathione.

Glutathione is a small protein composed of three amino acids. Amino acids are the building blocks of every part and system in the body. While we do create glutathione naturally from a variety of foods, the level that can be achieved solely from daily food intake is not enough to supply the demands created by drug toxins. Glutathione is the master anti-oxidant in the body, directly involved with detoxification. Glutathione binds up toxins in the body, transforming them so they can be excreted. An ample supply of glutathione is constantly needed for it to do its job properly at maximum levels.

The human body must also have an ample supply of vitamin B6, vitamin B12, and folate in order to convert one amino acid into another, which leads to the natural production of glutathione within the cells. This is a naturally occurring process when B6, B12 and folate are present. The body does not need or require a glutathione supplement for this process.

Once the body receives and recognizes sufficient required basic nutrients, it will set about creating all the glutathione it needs. Lacking the correct nutrients, the immune system and many other body areas cannot effectively get the show on the road, so to speak. With a malfunctioning immune system, and toxins not being broken down and eliminated, your body will suffer even worse drug withdrawal side effects as your toxicity levels rise.

Aktivated Barley™

Power Barley formula's second ingredient is Aktivated Barley. (And no, Aktivated is not misspelled). Barley historically has been used by everyone from warring Romans, to Greek gladiators-in-training, to mothers giving this magical food to their babies. Aktivated Barley is barley which has been turned into a "super food" via a patented process that captures all of the barley's powerful nutrients and energy just before flowering. Capturing these vital nutrients before the bloom stage provides more of what makes barley the miracle food it is.

Aktivated Barley is an excellent, slow burning, good carbohydrate. Its slow burning allows for a continuous, balanced absorption of the nutrients contained in the powdered formulation.

An example of slowed absorption's effect would be eating a very sugary dessert or meal and then *not* experiencing the normal "sugar rush." Impeding the flood of sugar into the blood stream causes the lack of sugar rush.

Aktivated Barley provides almost complete assimilation and utilization of its nutrients, without requiring large volumes as well as being extremely rich in naturally occurring amino acids, protein and other nutrients.

Due to the rich nutritional basis of the products contained in the formula and the slow, balanced absorption, this product is essential to healthy rebuilding of cells on the most basic level. These reasons, among many qualify Aktivated Barley as a "super food."

Carrot

The third ingredient of this formula is carrot for several very simple reasons - most obviously that it tastes great. But carrot also provides an ample supply of minerals in, again, a form easy to absorb and assimilate. Vitamin A is the most powerful vitamin supplied by carrots, boosting the immune system and abundant with antioxidant properties, also closely tied to proper cellular development and maintenance. For these reasons, carrots go hand-in-hand with all the other nutrient dense, alkaline-based ingredients that have been combined in this product.

If Cymbalta has caused you to have fatigue, you will be using the Power Barley Formula during this program.

Probiotic Supreme

Clinical trials have shown that at least 18% of the people who have taken an antidepressant have Candida yeast overgrowth. Three possible side effects of Candida yeast overgrowth are *depression, weight gain and bloating*. If you have ever used an antibiotic, a birth control pill, or most other medications, you have immensely increased the chance of Candida yeast overgrowth.

Other symptoms of Candida yeast overgrowth include – fatigue, recurring infections, mental fog, headaches, sore throat, abdominal pain, muscle tension and pain, joint pain or swelling, as well as digestive issues, such as heartburn, indigestion and Irritable Bowel Syndrome (IBS).

You may have a Candida yeast overgrowth, you may not. Lowering the inflammation marker, IL-6, is the ultimate goal. What we have found is a pre-biotic and probiotic blend, Probiotic Supreme, that will help rid the body of Candida yeast overgrowth and more importantly, help reduce the level of IL-6 in the process.

RenewPro

To further lower the inflammation marker IL-6, remove toxins and supply the body with all natural amino acids, we use a product called RenewPro. A complete book could be written on RenewPro and what it does within the human body.

First, RenewPro contains an exceptional amount of the amino acid cysteine. Cysteine lowers IL-6 significantly.

RenewPro will greatly increase the intracellular levels of our master antioxidant glutathione. Glutathione will lower IL-6.

A protein called lactoferrin is higher in RenewPro than any other whey protein product. Lactoferrin lowers IL-6.

If you are lacking energy or feeling dull, RenewPro is a must.

RenewPro is a whey protein concentrate made from disease-free, pesticide-free, chemical-free, hormone treatment-free and natural grass pasture fed cows.

Ultimate Omega 3

Your body's need for the essential oil Omega 3 and its highly beneficial qualities have been well covered in the news. Studies by doctors and health researchers have clarified the differences "good" and "bad" fats and the necessity of goods fats, such as Omega 3, in our diets.

Omega 3 is an essential fatty acid naturally derived from various types of fish. The two key chemical components in Omega 3 are **EPA** (Eicosapentaenoic acid) and **DHA** (Docosahexanoic). Both of these compounds, essential to your body's health, are available in either capsule or liquid form.

EPA assists the workings of your brain and neurological system – the system encompassing your nerves. EPA enhances the electrical functions and communications between all the systems in your body, which your body relies on to function properly.

DHA helps build the brain structurally, and as such, is a much-needed nutrient for the correct brain formation during growth. Both EPA and DHA are critical compounds for a person on psychiatric medications, as these drugs strip the body of these compounds. With these compounds stripped from the body, the communications or electrical impulses from one nerve ending to another do not flow smoothly, but rather jump in all directions creating such things as "brain zaps," "fogginess," irritability, agitation, forgetfulness and more.

"SUPER FOODS" USED ON THE ROAD BACK PROGRAM

Psychiatric medications directly oppose your body's neurological system, evidenced by the side effects experienced from the Cymbalta, as well as those suffered when trying to withdraw from them. Because of this the most critical element, between the EPA and DHA, is the EPA.

The amount of EPA and DHA taken during your taper will directly affect how well, or how poorly, you do on The Road Back Program.

If you will be tapering off an anti-depressant, anti-psychotic, or ADHD medication, it is doubly important that you use the correct quantity and quality of Omega 3. Here is a simple test to try, if you already have Omega 3 at home. Check the back of the bottle under "nutritional facts." If the label states less than 180 mg. of EPA per capsule, that bottle is grossly insufficient for the requirements of this program.

That Omega 3 will be less than effective, because when tapering off anti-depressants, anti-psychotics or ADHD medications you will need about 3,000 mg. of EPA each day. Doing the math, you can see that with the bottle above, you would need to take approximately 17 capsules of Omega 3 per day in order to get the correct quantity for your taper. Additionally, it is imperative that the Omega 3 that you take is free of any toxins or heavy metals.

Because your body is hypersensitive due to the Cymbalta, any metals whatsoever, from any source, are enough to turn on many symptoms, such as headaches, extreme irritably, massive agitation and more. As you may already be experiencing these symptoms from the Cymbalta, you certainly do not want to add to, or increase, them.

Omega 3 fish oil, high in EPA, is critical to use during the Cymbalta taper. For all head symptoms.

Vitamin E

Vitamin E is commonly found in regular foods, such as vegetable oils, nuts, whole grains and leafy vegetables. As discussed earlier, though found in many foods consumed on a regular basis it is difficult, if not impossible, to derive the total Vitamin E needed from diet alone.

Further, pollution, fried foods, bad carbohydrates, drugs, birth control pills, hormone replacement therapy and so many other bad influences test the vitamin E that we do have in our bodies. Vitamin E is an anti-oxidant, a natural compound that protects the body from toxins, and also helps protect other anti-oxidants in the body from being destroyed. It further helps the body eliminate circulating toxins or poisons. When taking the Power Barley Formula or RenewPro, you are causing a mild detoxification process – a good thing. Vitamin E helps your body neutralize these toxins and as these toxins un-stick themselves you will start to feel better with more energy.

The components making a complete vitamin and distinguishing available vitamin E's are staggering, having filled volumes. This program assists a person off Cymbalta and in the process ensures there will be no drug/supplement interactions with our recommendations. Beyond the correct mixture of vitamin E lies the quality or purity of a natural vitamin E. Some forms of vitamin E will create higher plasma concentrations of vitamin E while other forms will create vitamin E in the tissue. While Vitamin E is an antioxidant the incorrect vitamin E can become an oxidant and cause inflammation.

The A.C. Grace Company has been manufacturing vitamin E for more than 46 years. We recommend their Unique E with mixed tocopherols because of their manufacturing process and purity of product.

CHAPTER 4

CYMBALTA SIDE EFFECTS DEFINED

Side Effects of Cymbalta

The psychiatric medications we are dealing with are classified as psychotropic – having ability or quality of altering emotions, perceptions, behaviors, and bodily functions – especially true of certain drugs.

This chapter lists many possible Cymbalta side effects experienced from either taking Cymbalta, or when trying to withdraw from Cymbalta. If you, or anyone you know, is taking Cymbalta the "real you" could well be buried under some of the following symptoms. But rest assured, no one has all of these side effects, and no single drug or combination of these drugs can produce all the side effects listed here.

You may know from experience that a single Cymbalta withdrawal side effect can be horrifying. And if you, or anyone you know, have ever had a bad withdrawal experience you would probably rather sign up for open-heart surgery without anesthesia than suffer those side effects again. And for this very reason, many people who have contacted The Road Back are gun shy at the very thought of withdrawing from medication. Before The Road Back Program you were faced with a quandary: suffer the Cymbalta side effects, or gut it out and suffer the side effects of withdrawal.

The Road Back Program eliminates these worries and concerns by reducing to almost zero the side effects of withdrawal, so that you can come off the Cymbalta smoothly and easily.

The following list is broken down into categories, covering the various areas of the body, such as the nervous system, lymph system, emotional and mental symptoms and so forth. These categories will make it easier for you to find the part of the body or system that you are interested in, or want to know more about.

In this list you will find many physical ailments and complaints, as well as emotional or mental symptoms that people experience every day because of a specific medical condition. These symptoms and ailments may be the reason that you started Cymbalta, or conversely, the Cymbalta may actually be causing the negative symptoms you are experiencing now.

This unknown catches almost everyone, doctor and patient alike, off guard. So the question that needs to be answered in order for you to proceed with The Road Back Program is: Are you dealing with a physical condition that needs to be treated medically or with a by-product symptom of the Cymbalta?

Getting Your Doctor's Approval

Because of the overload and damage potentially caused by Cymbalta, your body in general, and your immune system in particular, are in a weakened condition, and can thus leave you open to infections and disease. On the other hand, you may be taking prescription medications for actual physical conditions, which could be contra-indicated in terms of doing The Road Back Program. These could include blood thinners and heart medication, as well as clotting agents.

Products used in The Road Back Program include Omega 3 and Vitamin E, which could both be contra-indicated if taking heart medications or blood thinners. Additionally, some of the products contain naturally occurring, (not synthetic) high levels of Vitamin K, which could be contra-indicated if taking any type of blood clotting medication.

For these reasons, consult your doctor ***before*** starting any part of this program to sort out, or discover and correctly determine, whether you are a candidate for The Road Back Program.

After you have ruled out any real medical problem, you will know that if any strange symptom begins during The Road Back Program, you are most likely experiencing something caused by the Cymbalta. Such will be true for both emotional and physical symptoms.

SIDE EFFECTS OF CYMBALTA

GENERAL BODY

Dry Mouth - Less moisture in the mouth than is usual.

Increased Sweating - A large quantity of perspiration that is medically caused.

Allergy - Extreme sensitivity of body tissues triggered by substances in the air, drugs, or foods causing a variety of reactions such as sneezing, itching, asthma, hay fever, skin rashes, nausea and/or vomiting.

Asthenia - A physically weak condition.

Chest Pains - Severe discomfort in the chest caused by not enough oxygen going to the heart because of blood vessel narrowing or spasms.

Chills - Appearing pale while cold and shivering. Sometimes accompanied by fever.

Edema of Extremities - Abnormal swelling of body tissue caused by the collection of fluid.

Fall - Suddenly losing a normal standing upright position.

Fatigue - Loss of normal strength thus not able to do usual physical and mental activities.

Fever - Abnormally high body temperature, normal being 98.6 degrees Fahrenheit or 37 degrees Centigrade. Fever is a symptom of disease or disorder in the body. The body is affected by feeling hot, chilled, sweaty, weak and exhausted. If the fever goes too high or lasts too long, death can result.

Hot Flashes - Brief, abnormal enlargement of the blood vessels that causes a sudden heat sensation over the entire body. Sometimes experienced by menopausal women.

Influenza (Flu)-like Symptoms - Demonstrating irritation of the respiratory tract (organs of breathing) such as a cold, sudden fever, aches and pains, as well as feeling weak and seeking bed rest, which is similar to having the flu.

Leg Pain - A hurtful sensation in the legs caused by excessive stimulation of the nerve endings in the legs, resulting in extreme discomfort.

Malaise - The somewhat unclear feeling of discomfort when a person starts to feel sick.

Pain in Limb - Sudden, sharp and uncontrolled leg or arm discomfort.

Syncope - A short period of light-headedness or unconsciousness (black-out) also known as fainting, caused by lack of oxygen to the brain because of an interruption in blood flow to the brain.

Tightness of Chest - Mild or sharp discomfort, tightness or pressure in the chest area (anywhere between the throat and belly). The causes can be mild or seriously life-threatening because they include the heart, lungs and surrounding muscles.

CARDIOVASCULAR
(INVOLVING THE HEART AND THE BLOOD VESSELS)

Palpitation - Unusual and abnormal heartbeat that is sometimes irregular, but rapid, and forceful thumping or fluttering. It can be brought on by shock, excitement, exertion or medical stimulants. A person is normally unaware of his/her heartbeat.

Hypertension - High blood pressure, a symptom of disease in the blood vessels leading away from the heart. Hypertension is known as the "silent killer." The symptoms are usually not obvious; however, it can lead to damage to the heart, brain, kidneys and eyes, and can even lead to stroke and kidney failure.

Bradycardia - The heart rate is slowed from around 72 beats per minute, which is normal, to below 60 beats per minute in an adult.

Tachycardia - The heart rate speeds up to above 100 beats per minute in an adult. Normal adult heart rate average is 72 beats per minute.

ECG Abnormal - A test called an electrocardiogram (ECG) records the activity of the heart by measuring heartbeats as well as the position and size of the heart's four chambers. An ECG also measures whether there is damage to the heart and the effects of drugs or mechanical devices like a heart pacemaker. When the test is abnormal this means one or more of the following are present: heart disease, defects, beating too fast or too slow, disease of the blood vessels leading from the heart or the heart valves, and/or a past or impending heart attack.

Flushing - Skin all over the body turns red.

Varicose Veins - Unusually swollen veins near the surface of the skin that sometimes appear twisted and knotted, but always enlarged. They are called hemorrhoids when appearing around the rectum. The cause is attributed to hereditary weakness in the veins aggravated by obesity, pregnancy, pressure from standing, aging, etc. Severe cases may develop swelling in the legs, ankles and feet, eczema and/or ulcers in the affected areas.

GASTROINTESTINAL
(INVOLVING THE STOMACH AND THE INTESTINES)

Abdominal Cramp/Pain - Sudden, severe, uncontrollable and painful shortening and thickening of the muscles in the belly. The belly includes the stomach, as well as the intestines, liver, kidneys, pancreas, spleen, gall bladder and urinary bladder.

Belching - Noisy release of gas from the stomach through the mouth; a burp.

Bloating - Swelling of the belly caused by excessive intestinal gas.

Constipation - Difficulty in having a bowel movement where the material in the bowels is hard due to a lack of exercise, fluid intake, or roughage in the diet or due to certain drugs.

Diarrhea - Unusually frequent and excessive runny bowel movements that may result in severe dehydration and shock.

Dyspepsia/Indigestion - The discomfort one may experience after eating. Can be heartburn, gas, nausea, a bellyache or bloating.

Flatulence - More gas than normal in the digestive organs.

Gagging - Involuntary choking and/or involuntary vomiting.

Gastritis - A severe irritation of the mucus lining of the stomach, either short in duration or lasting for a long period of time.

Gastroenteritis - A condition in which the membranes of the stomach and intestines are irritated.

Gastrointestinal Hemorrhage - Excessive internal bleeding in the stomach and intestines.

Gastro Esophageal Reflux - A continuous state where stomach juices flow back into the throat causing acid indigestion and heartburn and possibly injury to the throat.

Heartburn - A burning pain in the area of the breastbone caused by stomach juices flowing back up into the throat.

Hemorrhoids - Small rounded purplish swollen veins that bleed, itch or are painful and appear around the anus.

Increased Stool Frequency - see "Diarrhea."

Indigestion - Inability to properly consume and absorb food in the digestive tract, causing constipation, nausea, stomachache, gas, swollen belly, pain and general discomfort or sickness.

Nausea - Stomach irritation with a queasy sensation similar to motion sickness and a feeling that one is going to vomit.

Polyposis Gastric - Tumors that grow on stems in the lining of the stomach, which usually become cancerous.

Swallowing Difficulty - A feeling that food is stuck in the throat or upper chest area and won't go down, making it difficult to swallow.

Toothache - Pain in a tooth above and below the gum line.

Vomiting - Involuntarily throwing up the contents of the stomach, usually accompanied by a nauseated, sick feeling just prior to doing so.

HEMIC & LYMPHATIC
(INVOLVING THE BLOOD AND THE CLEAR FLUIDS IN THE TISSUES THAT CONTAIN WHITE BLOOD CELLS)

Anemia - A condition in which the blood is no longer carrying enough oxygen, so the person looks pale and easily gets dizzy, weak and tired. More severely, a person can end up with an abnormal heart, as well as breathing and digestive difficulties.

Bruise - Damage to the skin resulting in a purple-green-yellow skin coloration that is caused by breaking of the blood vessels in the area without breaking the surface of the skin.

Nosebleed - Blood loss from the nose.

Hematoma - Broken blood vessels that cause a swelling in an area on the body.

Lymphadenopathy Cervical - The lymph nodes in the neck, part of the body's immune system, become swollen and enlarged by reacting to the presence of a drug. The swelling is the result of the white blood cells multiplying in order to fight the invasion of the drug.

METABOLIC & NUTRITIONAL **(ENERGY AND HEALTH)**

Arthralgia - Sudden sharp nerve pain in one or more joints.

Arthropathy - Joint disease or abnormal joints.

Arthritis - Painfully inflamed and swollen joints. The reddened and swollen condition is brought on by a serious injury or shock to the body either from physical or emotional causes.

Back Discomfort - Severe physical distress in the area from the neck to the pelvis along the backbone.

Bilirubin Increased - Bilirubin is a waste product of the breakdown of old blood cells. Bilirubin is sent to the liver to be made water-soluble so it can be eliminated from the body through emptying the bladder. A drug can interfere with or damage this normal liver function, creating liver disease.

Decreased Weight - Uncontrolled and measured loss of heaviness or weight.

Gout - A severe arthritis condition that is caused by the dumping of a waste product called uric acid into the tissues and joints. It can worsen and cause the body to develop a deformity after going through stages of pain, inflammation, severe tenderness and stiffness.

Hepatic Enzymes Increased - An increase in the amount of paired liver proteins that regulate liver processes causing a condition in which the liver functions abnormally.

Hypercholesterolemia - Too much cholesterol in the blood cells.

Hyperglycemia - An unhealthy amount of sugar in the blood.

Increased Weight - A concentration and storage of fat in the body accumulating over a period of time caused by unhealthy eating patterns, a lack of physical activity, or an inability to process food correctly, which can predispose the body to many disorders and diseases.

Jaw Pain - Pain due to irritation and swelling of the nerves associated with the mouth area where it opens and closes just in front of the ear. Some of the symptoms are: pain when chewing, headaches, loss of balance, stuffy ears or ringing in the ears and teeth grinding.

Jaw Stiffness - The result of squeezing and grinding the teeth while asleep that can cause teeth to deteriorate, as well as the muscles and joints of the jaw.

Joint Stiffness - A loss of free motion and easy flexibility where any two bones come together.

Muscle Cramp - When muscles contract uncontrollably without warning and do not relax. The muscles of any body organs can cramp.

Muscle Stiffness - The tightening of muscles making it difficult to bend.

Muscle Weakness - Loss of physical strength.

Myalgia - A general widespread pain and tenderness of the muscles.

Thirst - A strong, unnatural craving for moisture/water in the mouth and throat.

NERVOUS SYSTEM (SENSORY CHANNELS)

Carpal Tunnel Syndrome - A pinched nerve in the wrist that causes pain, tingling, and numbing.

Coordination Abnormal - A lack of normal, harmonious interaction of the parts of the body when it is in motion.

Dizziness - Losing one's balance while feeling unsteady and lightheaded. May lead to fainting.

Disequilibrium - Lack of mental and emotional balance.

Faintness - A temporary condition in which one is likely to become unconscious and fall.

Headache - A sharp or dull persistent pain in the head

Hyperreflexia - A not normal (abnormal) and involuntary increased response in the tissues connecting the bones to the muscles.

Light-Headed Feeling - An uncontrolled and usually brief loss of consciousness usually caused by a lack of oxygen to the brain.

Migraine - Recurring severe head pain sometimes accompanied by nausea, vomiting, dizziness, flashes or spots before the eyes and ringing in the ears.

Muscle Contractions Involuntary - A spontaneous and uncontrollable tightening reaction of the muscles caused by electrical impulses from the nervous system.

Muscular Tone Increased - Uncontrolled and exaggerated muscle tension. Muscles are normally partially tensed which is what gives muscle tone.

Paresthesia - Burning, prickly, itchy, or tingling skin with no obvious or understood physical cause.

Restless Legs - A need to move the legs without any apparent reason. Sometimes there is pain, twitching, jerking, cramping, burning or a creepy-crawly sensation associated with the movements. It worsens when a person is inactive, and can interrupt sleep so one feels the need to move to gain some relief.

Shaking - Uncontrolled quivering and trembling as if one is cold and chilled.

Sluggishness - Lack of alertness and energy, as well as being slow to respond or perform in life.

Tics - A contraction of a muscle causing a repeated movement not under the control of the person, usually on the face or limbs.

Tremor - A nervous and involuntary vibrating or quivering of the body.

Twitching - Sharp, jerky and spastic motion, sometimes with a sharp sudden pain.

Vertigo - A sensation of dizziness with disorientation and confusion.

MENTAL AND EMOTIONAL

Aggravated Nervousness - A progressively worsening, irritated, and troubled state of mind.

Agitation - A suddenly violent and forceful emotionally disturbed state of mind.

Amnesia - Long or short term, partial or full memory loss created by emotional or physical shock, severe illness, or a blow to the head where the person was caused pain and became unconscious.

Anxiety Attack - Sudden and intense feelings of fear, terror, and dread, physically creating shortness of breath, sweating, trembling and heart palpitations.

Apathy - Complete lack of concern or interest for things that ordinarily would be regarded as important or would normally cause concern.

Appetite Decreased - Lack of appetite despite the ordinary caloric demands of living, with a resulting unintentional loss of weight.

Appetite Increased - An unusual hunger causing one to overeat.

Auditory Hallucination - Hearing things without the voices or noises being present.

Bruxism - Grinding and clenching of teeth while sleeping.

Carbohydrate Craving - A drive or craving to eat foods rich in sugar and starches (sweets, snacks and junk foods) that intensifies as the diet becomes more and more unbalanced due to the unbalancing of the proper nutritional requirements of the body.

Concentration Impaired - Unable to easily focus attention for long periods of time.

Confusion - Inability to think clearly or understand, preventing logical decision making.

Crying (Abnormal) - Unusual fits of weeping for short or long periods of time for no apparent reason.

Depersonalization - A condition in which one has lost a normal sense of personal identity.

Depression - A hopeless feeling of failure, loss and sadness that can deteriorate into thoughts of death. A very common reaction to or side effect of psychiatric drugs.

Disorientation - A loss of sense of direction, place, time or surroundings, as well as mental confusion regarding one's personal identity.

Dreaming (Abnormal) - Dreaming that leaves a very clear, detailed picture and impression when awake that can last for a long period of time and sometimes be unpleasant.

Emotional Lability - Suddenly breaking out in laughter or crying or doing both without being able to control the outburst of emotion. These episodes are unstable as they are caused by experiences or events that normally would not have this effect on an individual.

Excitability - Uncontrollably responding to stimuli (one's environment).

Feeling Unreal - The awareness that one has an undesirable emotion like fear, but can't seem to shake off the irrational feeling. For example, feeling like one is going crazy, but rationally knowing that it is not true. Resembles experiencing a bad dream and not being able to wake up.

Forgetfulness - Unable to remember what one ordinarily would remember.

Insomnia - Sleeplessness caused by physical stress, mental stress or stimulants, such as coffee or medications; a condition of being abnormally awake when one would ordinarily be able to fall and remain asleep.

Irritability - An abnormal reaction of being annoyed or disturbed in response to a stimulus in the environment.

Jitteriness - Nervous fidgeting without apparent cause.

Lethargy - Mental and physical sluggishness and *apathy* (a feeling of hopelessness that "nothing can be done") which can deteriorate into an unconscious state resembling deep sleep. A numbed state of mind.

Libido Decreased - An abnormal loss of sexual energy or desire.

Panic Reaction - A sudden, overpowering, chaotic and confused mental state of terror resulting in being doubt-ridden, often accompanied with *hyperventilation* and extreme anxiety.

Restlessness Aggravated - A constantly worsening troubled state of mind characterized by increased nervousness, inability to relax and quick temper.

Somnolence - Feeling sleepy all the time or having a condition of semi-consciousness.

Suicide Attempt - An unsuccessful deliberate attack on one's own life with the intention of ending it.

Suicidal Tendency - Most likely will attempt to kill oneself.

Tremulousness Nervous - Very jumpy, shaky, and uneasy, while feeling fearful and timid. The condition is characterized by dread of the future, involuntary quivering, trembling, and feeling distressed and suddenly upset.

Yawning - Involuntary opening of the mouth with deep inhalation of air.

REPRODUCTIVE FEMALE

Breast Neoplasm - A tumor or cancer, of either of the two milk-secreting organs on the chest of a woman.

Menorrhagia - Abnormally heavy menstrual period or a menstrual flow that has continued for an unusually long period of time.

Menstrual Cramps - Painful, involuntary uterus contractions that women experience around the time of their menstrual period, sometimes causing pain in the lower back and thighs.

Menstrual Disorder - A disturbance or derangement in the normal function of a woman's menstrual period.

Pelvic Inflammation - The reaction of the body to infectious, allergic or chemical irritation, which, in turn, causes tissue irritation, injury, or bacterial infection characterized by pain, redness, swelling, and sometimes loss of function. The reaction usually begins in the uterus and spreads to the fallopian tubes, ovaries and other areas in the hipbone region of the body.

Premenstrual Syndrome - Various physical and mental symptoms commonly experienced by women of childbearing age usually 2 to 7 days before the start of their monthly period. There are over 150 symptoms including eating binges, behavioral changes, moodiness, irritability, fatigue, fluid retention, breast tenderness, headaches, bloating, anxiety and depression.

The symptoms cease shortly after the period begins and disappear with menopause.

Spotting Between Menses - Abnormal bleeding between periods. Unusual spotting between menstrual cycles.

RESPIRATORY SYSTEM (ORGANS INVOLVED IN BREATHING)

Asthma - A disease of the breathing system initiated by an allergic reaction or a chemical, with repeated attacks of coughing, sticky mucus, wheezing, shortness of breath and a tight feeling in the chest. The disease can reach a state where it stops a person from exhaling, leading to unconsciousness and death.

Breath Shortness - Unnatural breathing, using a lot of effort resulting in not enough air taken in by the body.

Bronchitis - Inflammation of the two main breathing tubes leading from the windpipe to the lungs. The disease is marked by coughing, a low-grade fever, chest pain and hoarseness. Can also be caused by an allergic reaction.

Coughing - A cough is the response to an irritation, such as mucus, that causes the muscles controlling the breathing process to expel air from the lungs suddenly and noisily to keep the air passages free from the irritating material.

Laryngitis - Inflammation of the voice box characterized by hoarseness, sore throat, and coughing. It can be caused by straining the voice or exposure to infectious, allergic or chemical irritation.

Nasal Congestion - The presence of an abnormal amount of fluid in the nose.

Pneumonia Tracheitis - Bacterial infection of the air passageways and lungs that causes redness, swelling and pain in the windpipe. Other symptoms are high fever, chills, pain in the chest, difficulty breathing and coughing with mucus discharge.

Rhinitis - Chemical irritation causing pain, redness and swelling in the mucus membranes of the nose.

Sinus Congestion - The mucus-lined areas of the bones in the face that are thought to help warm and moisten air to the nose. These areas become clogged with excess fluid or become infected.

Sinus Headache - An abnormal amount of fluid in the hollows of the facial bone structure, especially around the nose. This excess fluid creates pressure, causing pain in the head.

Sinusitis - The body reacting to chemical irritation causing redness, swelling and pain in the area of the hollows in the facial bones especially around the nose.

SKELETAL

Neck/Shoulder Pain - Hurtful sensations of the nerve endings caused by damage to the tissues in the neck and shoulder, signaling danger of disease.

SKIN AND APPENDAGES (SKIN, LEGS AND ARMS)

Acne - Eruptions of the oil glands of the skin, especially on the face, marked by pimples, blackheads, whiteheads, bumps and more severely, by cysts and scarring.

Alopecia - The loss of hair, baldness.

Angioedema - Intense itching and swelling welts on the skin called hives caused by an allergic reaction to internal or external agents. The reaction is common to a food or a drug. Chronic cases can last for a long period of time.

Dermatitis - Generally irritated skin that can be caused by any of a number of irritating conditions, such as parasites, fungus, bacteria, or foreign substances causing an allergic reaction. It is a general inflammation of the skin.

Dry Lips - The lack of normal moisture in the fleshy folds that surround the mouth.

Dry Skin - The lack of normal moisture/oils in the surface layer of the body. The skin is the body's largest organ.

Epidermal Necrolysis - An abnormal condition in which a large portion of the skin becomes intensely red and peels off like a second-degree burn. Symptoms often include blistering.

Eczema - A severe or continuing skin disease marked by redness, crusting and scaling, with watery blisters and itching. It is often difficult to treat and will sometimes go away only to reappear again.

Folliculitis - Inflammation of a follicle (small body sac), especially a hair follicle. A hair follicle contains the root of a hair.

Furunculosis - Skin boils that show up repeatedly.

Lipoma - A tumor of mostly fat cells that is not health endangering.

Pruritus - Extreme itching of often-undamaged skin.

Rash - A skin eruption or discoloration that may or may not be itching, tingling, burning or painful. It may be caused by an allergy, a skin irritation or a skin disease.

Skin Nodule - A bulge, knob, swelling or outgrowth in the skin that is a mass of tissue or cells.

RELATED TO THE SENSES

Conjunctivitis - Infection of the membrane that covers the eyeball and lines the eyelid, caused by a virus, allergic reaction or an irritating chemical. It is characterized by redness, a discharge of fluid and itching.

Dry Eyes - Not enough moisture in the eyes.

Earache - Pain in the ear.

Eye Infection - The invasion of the eye tissue by a bacteria, virus, fungus, etc, causing damage to the tissue, with toxicity. Infection spreading in the body progresses into disease.

Eye Irritation - An inflammation of the eye.

Metallic Taste - A range of taste impairment from distorted taste to a complete loss of taste.

Pupils Dilated - Abnormal expansion of the black circular opening in the center of the eye.

Taste Alteration - Abnormal flavor detection in food.

Tinnitus - A buzzing, ringing or whistling sound in one or both ears occurring from the use of certain drugs.

Vision Abnormal - Normal images are seen differently by the viewer than by others.

Vision Blurred - Eyesight is dim or indistinct and hazy in outline or appearance.

Visual Disturbance - Eyesight is interfered with or interrupted. Examples of disturbances are light sensitivity and the inability to easily distinguish colors.

URINARY SYSTEM

Blood in Urine - Blood is present when one empties the liquid waste product of the kidneys through the bladder by urinating in the toilet, turning the water pink to bright red. Or spots of blood are observable in the water after urinating.

Dysuria - Difficult or painful urination.

Kidney Stone - Small hard masses of salt deposits that the kidney forms.

Urinary Frequency - Having to urinate more often than usual or between unusually short time periods.

Urinary Tract Infection - An invasion of bacteria, viruses, fungi, etc., of the system in the body. This starts with the kidneys, which eliminate urine from the body. If the invasion goes unchecked, it can injure tissue and progress into disease.

Urinary Urgency - A sudden compelling urge to urinate, accompanied by discomfort in the bladder.

UROGENITAL **(URINARY TRACT AND/OR GENITAL STRUCTURES OR FUNCTIONS)**

Anorgasmia - Failure to experience an orgasm.

Ejaculation Disorder - Dysfunction of the discharge of semen during orgasm.

Menstrual Disorder - Dysfunction of the discharge during the monthly menstrual cycle.

VIOLENT OR PHYSICALLY DANGEROUS SIDE EFFECTS

Acute Renal Failure - The kidneys stop excreting waste products properly, leading to rapid poisoning (toxicity) in the body.

Anaphylaxis - A violent, sudden, and severe drop in blood pressure caused by a re-exposure to a foreign protein or a second dosage of a drug that may be fatal unless emergency treatment is given right away.

Grand Mal Seizures (or Convulsions) - A recurring sudden, violent and involuntary attack of muscle spasms with a loss of consciousness.

Neuroleptic Malignant Syndrome - A life threatening, rare reaction to an anti-psychotic drug marked by fever, muscular rigidity, changed mental status and dysfunction of the autonomic nervous system.

Pancreatitis - Chemical irritation with redness, swelling and pain in the pancreas where digestive enzymes and hormones are secreted.

QT Prolongation - A very fast heart rhythm disturbance that is too fast for the heart to beat effectively so the blood to the brain falls, causing a sudden loss of consciousness. May cause sudden cardiac arrest.

Rhabdomyolysis - The breakdown and release of muscle fibers into the circulatory system. Some of the fibers are poisonous to the kidney and frequently result in kidney damage.

Serotonin Syndrome - A disorder brought on by excessive levels of *serotonin*. Caused by drugs and can be fatal. Symptoms include euphoria, drowsiness, sustained and rapid eye movement, agitation, reflexes overreacting, rapid muscle contractions, abnormal movements of the foot, clumsiness, feeling drunk and dizzy without any intake of alcohol, jaw muscles contracting and relaxing excessively, muscle twitching, high body temperature, rigid body, rotating mental status - including confusion and excessive happiness - diarrhea and loss of consciousness.

Thrombocytopenia - An abnormal decrease in the number of blood platelets in the circulatory system. A decrease in platelets causes a decrease in the ability of the blood to clot when necessary.

Torsades de Pointes - Unusually rapid heart rhythm starting in the lower heart chambers. If the short bursts of rapid heart rhythm continue for a prolonged period, it can degenerate into a more rapid rhythm and can be fatal.

CHAPTER 5

THINGS TO BE AWARE OF

There are several medical situations you need to be aware of before you start this program. First let me repeat, check with your doctor before starting this program. Medically and physically, do this for your health and safety as you travel though this process.

I understand there could be a problem: possibly your doctor does not support tapering off the medication.

In such a case, check The Road Back website *www.theroadback.org* or call us at 1-866-892-0238. We constantly add to our list of doctors who endorse and use The Road Back Program to help their patients taper off psychiatric medications. You can also find doctors more integrative in their approach to medicine and its application in helping patients heal. These doctors have a broader view of medicine, a greater understanding of how nutritional support relates to the body or would be open to and/or schooled in different healing methods.

This is your journey. Find those who will help you travel the proven successful road laid out for you.

Physical Conditions and Drug Interactions

Many people have contacted me over the years, asking about their activities and/or medications taken and whether they can use these in combination with The Road Back Program. My answer? Check with your doctor about medications and how these could interact with other supplements, vitamins, drugs and so on. Having said that, I know various medical conditions and/or drugs could possibly interfere with this program, including the following:

1. **Blood thinners and heart medication**

    Omega 3 and Vitamin E both thin the blood. Taking either of these supplements, in conjunction with a medication that is already thinning your blood, could be contra-indicated, or not advised. This is for your doctor to determine.

2. **Clotting agents**

    Some of the supplements used on The Road Back contain naturally high levels of Vitamin K. This vitamin has clotting and healing properties, and as such, could create additional clotting that would not be beneficial. Again, this is for your doctor to determine

Alternative Therapies

While I have personally seen the results from natural health and healing practices, each has its own purpose and end result. Additionally, I have found they can too often can be counterproductive when used in conjunction with The Road Back Program. Any alternative therapy or health practice that recommends additional nutrients, supplements, vitamins, drips, sprays, drinks and methodologies can and do exacerbate, aggravate or make worse, the very sensitive process we are trying to guide you through now.

Due to the Cymbalta, your system is essentially balanced on the "head of a pin," meaning that your tolerance for *anything* can be, or is, very limited.

The Road Back Program has been researched and developed around very specific parameters, undercutting any other health products. While these other health products might be great in a healthy, balanced body, they often do not mix well with psychiatric medications and your tapering process. Right now you need to slowly and safely taper off your medications. Add other health products back into your daily regime after you have completed this venture. Once completely and safely off these medications, by all means, help yourself.

While on The Road Back Program taking various health products adds one more thing to an already overloaded system. Therefore, I emphatically recommend you evaluate these alternative therapies, practices, nutritional items and restrict them until successfully completing your program.

Specifically, anything that moves medications too rapidly through your body should be avoided.

Remember, "Slow and steady wins the race."

CHAPTER 6

GENERAL PRE-TAPERING AND TAPERING INSTRUCTIONS

Despite apparent redundancy, what I am about to say cannot be said too many times, so bear with me.

As you start your road back, I want your journey to be as successful and as smooth as possible. Therefore I repeat; *you cannot simply quit Cymbalta cold turkey.*

You must methodically taper off Cymbalta, giving your body all possible assistance to ensure you fully complete this program and are not driven back onto your prescriptions.

Your program consists of a two-part process: First, the pre-taper, which averages three weeks. The three week time period is not exact; it varies for each individual. That's fine as this is not a race against the clock. This is a journey back to you through steady steps that become more and more certain over time.

Once finished with the pre-taper, you will start the actual taper. You will start to reduce the Cymbalta while continuing your "super foods" and supplements. The number of medications you are currently taking, and your speed of progress each step along the way, will determine the length of the tapering process.

This chapter is an overview of the pre-tapering and tapering process, and what you will do no matter which drug or drugs you are taking.

These steps are vitally important to your success. Please study them carefully to ensure confidence when beginning your personal program.

The Purpose of the Pre-Taper

Just as in running a marathon, swimming a mile, buying a house, or having a baby, you have to build up to the ultimate goal. The same applies with The Road Back Program. You need to stretch your muscles, get some good nutrition into your system and know how your daily schedule will change. The Pre Taper will set you up for a smooth reduction off Cymbalta. This will be a period of gradual adjustment allowing you to ease into the program and to see how it goes.

Do not underestimate this first step, as it has its own goals, victories and discoveries. A few milestones must be reached before moving fully onto the reduction of your particular medications.

The Pre-Taper Goals

- Elimination, or a *drastic* reduction, of all existing side effects caused by the Cymbalta.

- Determining which "super foods" and supplements created the positive change.

  When you know the exact supplement or "super food" in the pre-taper that eliminated the side effects, you will know how to eliminate that side effect, if it recurs during the reduction phase of your program.

The reasoning: If a withdrawal side effect begins during the taper, odds are that it was one of the existing side effects you had *before you started your pre-taper*.

GENERAL PRE-TAPERING AND TAPERING INSTRUCTIONS

An example of the importance of the pre-taper is found in the Introduction to *The Art of War* by Sun Tzu, from Thomas Cleary's translation.

"Plan for what is difficult while it is easy, do what is great while it is small. The most difficult things in the world must be done while they are still easy; the greatest things in the world must be done while they are still small."

Nutritional Supplements

Review the Chapter "Super Foods Used on The Road Back Program" and make sure you have the "super foods" and nutritional supplements on hand. The day before you start your pre-taper, review which supplements you will be taking the next day, and the times you will be taking them. If you will be carrying the "super foods" and supplements with you during the day, and need to put those quantities into smaller containers, do so. If you know that you have a busy schedule on the day that you will start, or any day following that, prepare by making a note of when you need to take your supplements and how you can arrange to do so. If you do not usually carry water with you, or have it available where you will be, take some with you.

As stated earlier, this program is a work in progress. We constantly research better ways to eliminate side effects and speed up the tapering process.

This edition is required due to recent breakthroughs. Today a person can taper completely off their medication in half the time previously required.

The changes to the program are additional supplements that directly target specific areas of the immune system which we know will be either too high or too low, depending on side effects or medication being used. The ability to pinpoint exact areas of the body with these new supplements has more rapidly eliminated anxiety, depression, fatigue and a host of other side effects.

You can still follow the slower method of tapering off medication if you or your physician desires that approach.

Your Daily Journal:

Every day you will keep a written record of your progress in a journal.

Review the chapter "Daily Journal." You are free to copy the journal and put together your own, or you can find pre-made journals at The Road Back website. In your Daily Journal you will note certain information over the course of a 24-hour period. These specific statistics are important because they will help you find your way back to center, if you falter at any point during the program. Before going to bed each night, or during the day as you take each step, write down the following:

- The date.
- The time of all medications you took that day and dosage amount.
- All food and drinks, including coffee, water, alcohol, etc; times you ate or drank, and the amount.
- Rate your own progress as to how you feel.
- Rate your energy, appetite, mood and exercise.
- Include anything that you added or deleted from your daily routine.

Keeping the journal allows you to review changes and determine which ones made positive improvements. But if a problem occurs, the journal allows you to look back and locate which change may have made a negative impact. Locating such will enable you to quickly fix what changed and get yourself back on track.

For example, you may have increased your supplements and "super foods" too quickly or too much, and now you need to reduce them to the quantity you were taking when you last felt good. Or possibly you felt so good from the pre-taper that you added exercise into your day, which created a negative change. Whatever the case, it could be a small and seemingly insignificant change, or it could be a major change that you did not realize you had made. Using your Daily Journal, you will be able to find your way back. The Daily Journal will act like a positive voice sitting on your shoulder reminding you of what works for you, and what does not.

By noting the exact quantity of each supplement you have taken daily, you will know the positive changes are a direct result of the exact amounts and times you took your "super foods" and supplements.

The Following Is Key to Your Success:

If emotions, physical complaints, energy, mood or anything else improves, you will remain at the same intake level of the supplement or "super food" that created the improvement. You will be introducing each "super food" or supplement slowly. Once you experience a positive change with any "super food" or supplement, continue the amount that caused the positive change. By keeping a record, you will be able to quickly chart your improvement while moving through the pre-taper and tapering programs. Your journal will become a critical ally in your journey, helping you helm your ship and master your destiny.

Make sure you use your Daily Journal to track your progress.

Recreational Drugs and Alcohol

There might not be a lot to say on this subject that you do not already know. Firstly, either of these items, recreational drugs and/or alcohol, can create or bring on unwanted physical symptoms during your tapering process. Use of either could also cause or contribute to existing problems, mask potential problems, or aggravate problems that already exist. While I have said do not change anything you are doing in your life, this is one area where that adage does not apply. Completing The Road Back Program *is not* about "having your cake and eating it too."

Becoming medication-and-symptom-free is your goal. Give yourself the chance to accomplish your goal.

Do Not Change Anything

Since I just told you to stop taking recreational drugs and alcohol, I might now seem to be contradicting myself, but not so.

For example: If you are already on some form of exercise program, and starting The Road Back Program, you would not stop exercising. It is great for your body, and *your* body is: used to this routine.

If not on an exercise program, do not suddenly start because it seems like a good idea in combination with the tapering process. Your body is not ready for both these changes at the same time and there could be hell to pay. However, you can go for a slow, casual walk daily if you wish. That is fine and recommended.

Also note the following:

- Do not start a liver-cleansing process, colon cleanse, etc. and the taper at the same time.

- Do not stop drinking coffee, smoking or abruptly change your diet and start this program at the same time.

Each one of these dos and don'ts: a) has its own chemical response in your system and b) any of these can either speed up or slow down the flow of medications you are taking through your body, and thus could create withdrawal side effects.

While some supplements are good for you and some supplements may not be as beneficial, it will be too hard to sort out what causes what, therefore you may find it difficult to keep yourself on a steady path gaining momentum and success. You get the point – use your head. Examine the options and choose the one that adheres as closely to The Road Back Program as possible.

GENERAL PRE-TAPERING AND TAPERING INSTRUCTIONS

Deviation from The Road Back Program

You might think deviating from the program would be the obvious and easy to detect. Not always.

The Road Back Program usually works quickly; the person quickly experiencing a vast improvement. This blessing can also be a curse. In the first years of the program, a person would typically feel a major positive change about half-way through the tapering portion. Now they frequently experience major positive change after a few days on the pre-taper. The creation of the "super foods" and the time of day each is taken have greatly sped up the program. Imagine feeling as though you had never taken a drug only one week after starting the pre-taper part of The Road Back Program.

However, when this major positive change occurs, a person can feel so good that he or she begins doing things they have wanted to do for years, such as quitting smoking, giving up coffee or starting a major exercise program.

Then they suddenly crash and wonder why!

I first experienced this curse in 1999 when a woman called who was tapering off her medication. After first doing well, suddenly she was not. She had tried to taper off antidepressant medication several times over the years before starting The Road Back Program, never reducing the drug without extreme withdrawal and always returning to her original dosage. This time she had been half-way off her medication and feeling great.

It took two weeks to figure out what changed. I asked every question I could think of; there was something she was doing differently. I finally found out that typically, every six months, she went onto an all-protein diet. This was so "normal" for her she never thought to mention, or view it, as a major change in her lifestyle. However, this diet change hugely impacted her progress, and _was_ the major deviation from the program. Once the change was discovered, she re-started her tapering program from square one and successfully completed.

I cannot over stress looking for and finding obvious as well as subtle changes if you experience a negative change during this program.

Another major deviation from the program can occur – you feel so good, you forget to take your medication(s). This is a no-no, but happens. Lower the medication only at specific amounts and make that gradual reduction. Numerous people over the years have begun a pre-taper while suffering from widely varying side effects. Taking psychiatric medications for years, they had tried to get off the drugs countless times. After beginning the pre-taper and finally sleeping through the night for the first time in months, their daytime anxiety vanished. Three days later, they forgot to take their medication at bedtime. The next day, they went into full withdrawal and began to question whether The Road Back Program was right for them. The only problem was forgetting to take their medication.

These variations or deviations from the program can also be extremely troubling for a doctor. He or she can only help guide you through the steps with all the information on hand. Again, it is imperative that: a) you write everything down in your Daily Journal, including things you might think have no bearing whatsoever, and b) bring your Daily Journal to your doctor visits, so that together you can chart your progress and get back to square one if needed.

A Recommendation of
What to Add During or After the Program

Many of you are now suffering from anxiety and or depression as a medication side effect. You may have suffered from anxiety or depression before the medication and that is why you are now taking the drug you wish to taper.

If a person were to change anything or add anything to their daily routine while doing this program I recommend the Depression Recovery Program. Let's face it; if you did not have traumatic stress before the medication, you may now. Being medication free and medication side effect free is one major part of the battle, but being able to *fully* address the underlying causes, the things that might hold negative feelings, unwanted emotions and personal erratic considerations in place need to be resolved at some point in time.

You can and it is urged that you do begin this concurrently with the pre-taper. If that is not possible, certainly accomplish this once off the Cymbalta to achieve that lasting result.

Contact Depression Recovery Program at 1-785-594-7070 or www.depressionrecoveryprogram.org for more information.

"Super Foods"

A deviation from The Road Back Program can also take place with the "super foods" used on the program. Once you feel a positive change with the Power Barley Formula, do not increase it further during the pre-taper.

I often make this joke about Texans and Power Barley Formula. Big, or better yet bigger, is better in Texas. On a trip to Texas I described how to use the Power Barley Formula, what to look for regarding positive changes and to not increase that product once positive change is achieved.

Two weeks later, a Texan called raving about her positive changes. One week later, the same person called again, saying they did not feel as well and were wondering what could have happened. This was not too difficult to solve. Texans and Power Barley Formula? The person had doubled the Power Barley Formula amount that brought on the positive changes. If one teaspoon three times a day made you feel that good, 2 teaspoons 3 times a day should make you feel twice as good, was the thought process.

Once the Texan went back to the right amount for her body, she felt good again.

Major Improvement

The Texan story leads us to the definition of major change - a major improvement. A major improvement is what you are going for with the pre-taper.

If you have extreme daytime anxiety and are able to reduce it to a point where you have to stop and look for anxiety to even see or feel any, you have had a major improvement.

If you could not sleep more than two hours a night and are now able to sleep four to five hours, wake up and then go back to sleep, that is a major improvement.

If every joint in your body ached, and now you have only a little ache in the morning when you awake that goes away within the first few minutes, you have experienced a major improvement.

If you felt a major depression every day and now you feel a little depressed occasionally, you have had a major improvement.

If you feel like you are not even taking a medication now, you have had a major improvement.

Major changes are what you are going for during the pre-taper. The goal is to alleviate major complaints or reduce them to the point of being very acceptable and not in the way of day-to-day life, so that you can fully taper off the medication and "live life."

Once a "super food" or supplement provides relief or a major improvement, there is no need to keep *increasing* that product.

Steady State: The term "steady state" has special definitions in biochemistry, chemistry, electronics and even macroeconomics.

In The Road Back Program "steady state" is defined as: A constant level or a level of action that allows a balance between two or more substances.

A *constant level* would be maintaining a level of a supplement in the body to a degree where it never drops below a certain point. Much like the half-life of medication, keeping enough of a substance in the body at a specific strength gives a result. If you skip a dosage of medication, withdrawal begins. If you skip a serving of a supplement, withdrawal does not take place, but you do lose the steady or constant state of the supplement.

A *level of action that allows a balance between two or more substances* is different from a *constant level*. Psychiatric medications alter hormones and the adrenals. When a "steady state" occurs with the nutritionals at a *constant level*, the cells will use the nutrients to begin working with each other, balancing each other, allowing the cells to receive energy and exchange back to other cells desired substances for optimum survival.

During the pre-taper, one goal is finding the "steady state" of each nutritional for your body. Age, height, weight, gender, how long you have been using a medication or the type of medication you might be using *cannot* be used to predict the correct amount of a nutritional. This takes trial and success. This is one reason you begin each nutritional at a small amount and only increase the nutritional to the point of a positive change.

If You Have Anxiety or Insomnia, What to Expect

The following chart is the result of a double-blind randomized controlled trial of the benzodiazepine Oxazepam. Oxazepam is also marketed under the names Alepam, Murelax, Oxascand, Serax, Serepax, Seresta and Sobril.

The trial was for treatment of generalized anxiety.

Two groups were used. One group received Oxazepam plus a placebo while the other used Passion Flower and a placebo. The Body Calm Supreme used with The Road Back Program is the Passion Flower available closest to that used in the trial.

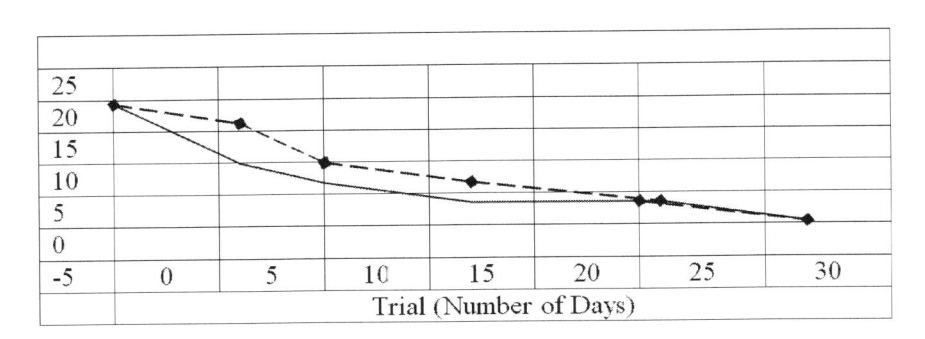

```
25
20
15
10
 5
 0
-5     0     5    10    15    20    25    30
              Trial (Number of Days)
```

—————— Oxazepam plus placebo
♦ — — — — ♦ Passion Flower plus placebo

Left Column is the Hamilton Anxiety Score.

Notice the gradual reduction of anxiety over 30 days. Use the graph located after the "Daily Journal" chapter to chart your own progress.

Calcium-Induced Side Effects With Benzodiazepines and Anti-Convulsants

Many of you may be taking a benzodiazepine as well as Cymbalta. For that reason we have included information regarding benzodiazepines.

- When taking benzodiazepines and/or anti-convulsants, do not take a supplement containing ionic calcium.

If you are taking an antidepressant or anti-psychotic medication and anxiety is a major complaint, avoid ionic calcium as well.

If you are going to take calcium, make sure to include 5 grams each day of Calsorption to improve the calcium absorption and ideally use a calcium product like CalesiumD.

Ionic calcium and "plain" or unaltered calcium differ in that ionic calcium is altered into a form the body absorbs instantly versus "plain" or unaltered calcium, which breaks down in the body more slowly. An ionic calcium product either dissolves or fizzes when put into hot or cold liquid.

While either type of calcium wonderfully supplements a natural, healthy diet, do not use ionic calcium if taking a benzodiazepine or if suffering from anxiety. Calcium is something all bodies require, and one main property is assisting with the correct functioning of nerve impulses. While you want your nerves and their impulses functioning correctly at all times, you do not want or need to increase or "feed" this nerve stimulation while you are taking and/or trying to taper off of benzodiazepines and/or anti-convulsants.

Calcium stimulates electrical discharge of the nerves. The stimulation of nerve impulses is the primary problem associated with using ionic calcium along with a benzodiazepine or anticonvulsant.

Clinical trials have shown that blocking calcium can help protect a person from the worst benzodiazepine withdrawal symptoms.

Calcium-induced side effects while taking a benzodiazepine or anti-convulsant can include:

- Hyperkinesia: an abnormal increase in muscular activity, hyperactivity, especially in children.

- Hyperthermia: unusually high body temperature.

- Hyper aggression.

- Audiogenic seizures: Seizures caused by loud sounds and noises.

- Increased anxiety.

- Psychosis.

- Numbness around the mouth.

- Tingling in the extremities.

- Shortness of breath.

It is vital that you ensure you are not taking an ionic calcium supplement while using a benzodiazepine or anti-convulsant.

Several patients and physicians have contacted The Road Back with questions about using calcium as part of The Road Back Program.

Suggestion: If you are taking a calcium supplement and suffer from anxiety, stop the calcium supplement for three days. See if the anxiety goes away or greatly subsides. If the anxiety subsides, there is nothing left to argue about. If the anxiety stays the same, it is not the calcium. Keep taking the calcium!

Your Next Step

- If you are taking a benzodiazepine, anti-convulsant, anti-anxiety or sleep medication, follow the instructions found in the chapter "Pre-Taper for Benzodiazepine, Anti-convulsant, Anti-anxiety, and Sleep Medication."

- If you are only taking Cymbalta, follow the instructions found in the chapter "Pre-Taper for Antidepressants, Anti-Psychotics, and ADHD Medication."

- If you are taking a benzodiazepine, anti-convulsant, anti-anxiety or sleep medication along with an antidepressant, anti-psychotic or ADHD medication follow the instructions found in the chapter "Pre-Taper for Antidepressants, Anti-Psychotics, and ADHD Medication." In that chapter, there is a section "If You Have Anxiety or Insomnia." Follow the pre-taper instructions in that section.

Two Key Components for Accomplishing a Complete and Successful Taper:

1. Fully complete your *pre-tapering* program before starting your medication- reduction tapering program.

2. Taper off the medication using the correct reduction amount to match your body. The book's chapters cover tapering off medication in two ways. One, a very slow and gradual reduction, with a chapter

title containing *Slow and Gradual Taper*. The other providing details to reduce the medication twice as fast using the all new approach and titled *Fast and Gradual Taper*.

Taking either of those two paths will tilt the scales in your favor. Both allow for a high degree of control over the process. I want you to have this control. These steps allow the body time to recover from drug effects, with the added benefit of rest and correct nutritional "super foods" and supplements.

CHAPTER 7

DAILY JOURNAL

Date: _____ Pre-Taper/Taper (Circle one)   Day # _____ Step # _____

Note: **<u>Do Not Change Eating or Exercise Habits During The Program!</u>**

Current Drugs & Dosages: (List all taken, time of day and amount)

_____ _____ _____ _____
_____ _____ _____ _____

Food and Liquid:
(List all food and liquid consumed, time of day and amount)

The Road Back Nutritionals: (List all taken, time of day and amount)

<u>**Rate the Following Areas Using a Scale of 1 to 10**</u>: (Rate daytime anxiety at bedtime and rate the previous night's sleep first thing in the morning. Rate all other items before bedtime.)

Symptom	**1-10 Rating**	**List All Changes Made During the Day**
Aches		
Anxiety		
Appetite		
Body Pains		
Energy		
Exercise		

Fatigue		
Mood		
Sleep		

CHAPTER 8

GRAPH YOUR SUCCESS

A graph for each symptom you are rating each day can greatly help tracking your progress and allow you to look back at how far you have come.

See an example below of how to fill in the graph. The next page is a blank graph for you to copy or recreate on your own.

Pre-Taper / Taper (Circle one)   Day   #   _____   Step   #   _____

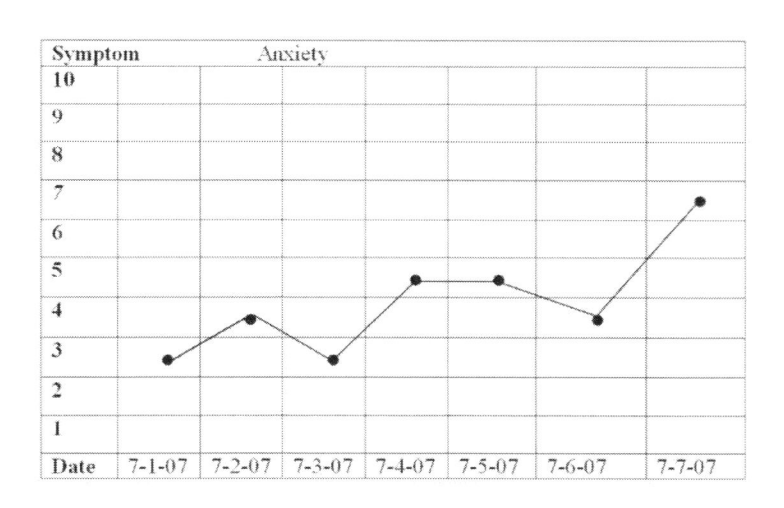

Symptom	Anxiety						
10							
9							
8							
7							●
6							
5				●	●		
4		●				●	
3	●		●				
2							
1							
Date	7-1-07	7-2-07	7-3-07	7-4-07	7-5-07	7-6-07	7-7-07

71

Notice the trend change beginning on the fourth. The trend continues the next day and then drops one day, but rebounds to a 7-rating on the last day of the week.

This is a normal daily trend during the beginning of the pre-taper. If you have already quit taking the medication and are suffering from withdrawal side effects, make sure you use these graphs. I understand you need hope, and seeing for yourself may spark the hope that inspires you to continue and make it back.

After graphing each day and symptom for a period of time, you will see a longer-term trend. Placing each graph side-by-side you can easily see your ratings for several weeks and your trend for each symptom.

Make sure you take your Daily Journal and graphs to your doctor visits.

By running each graph for seven days, you can attach one completed graph to seven days of your Daily Journal and create a weekly file.

Daily Graph

Symptom							
10							
9							
8							
7							
6							
5							
4							
3							
2							
1							
Date							

CHAPTER 9

PRE-TAPER FOR BENZODIAZEPINES, ANTI-ANXIETY, ANTICONVULSANTS AND SLEEP MEDICATION

"I am taking Klonopin. After one week on your program, I do not feel like I am taking a benzo. I am sleeping better than I ever have in my life. Vivid dreams have vanished and if I wake up in the middle of the night, I can go right back to sleep. I will be starting the taper next week and I am very nervous. Every time I have tried to quit in the past, the withdrawal was too much. Everything you have said in your book has been true so far so I probably should not be nervous."

G.Q.
Green Bay, WI.

Many people taking Cymbalta are also taking a benzodiazepine or sleep medication. You may be required to taper off the benzodiazepine or sleep medication before tapering off the Cymbalta and I do not want you to be forced to wait on the arrival of another book describing how to get off those medications. The chapters on benzodiazepines are general instructions for this class of medication but they instructions do apply to all benzodiazepines as well as to all sleep medications.

If you have not yet read the entire chapter "General Pre-Tapering and Tapering Guidelines," please do so before continuing with this chapter. Reading and understanding the "General Pre-Tapering and Tapering Guidelines" is *vital* before starting the pre-taper.

Starting Your Pre-Taper

Note: This pre-taper addresses several types of medication as noted in the chapter title. If the only drug named is a benzodiazepine, please take that to mean all medications (Benzodiazepine, *Anti-anxiety, Anticonvulsant and Sleep Medication*).

Physically, during the pre-taper and taper, you need to address a substance called Interleukin-2 (IL-2). A blood test can measure the level of IL-2 in your body. If a person has anxiety and/or insomnia their IL-2 levels will be too low. IL-2 is part of the human immune system.

There are several things that might have made your IL-2 too low initially. If you work in an office building, installed new carpet at home or in the office, you are probably breathing positive air ions, instead of negative. Positive air ions will lower the body's IL-2 levels and create an anxiety feeling. Increase the IL-2 level in your body as slowly and naturally as possible.

The air you breathe is not the only cause of IL-2 reduction, but if walking at night, walking after rain or standing by a waterfall drops your anxiety levels, it might be because negative air ions were just in your proximity. No running out and purchasing an air ionizer, they do not fix what really needs to be handled with air quality.

IL-2 levels are objectively tested. You and your physician can work on those levels to treat your anxiety and insomnia. Stage 2 of sleep (deep night sleep) requires ample amount of IL-2. Read additional information about IL-2 in the chapter, The Science Behind The Road Back.

PRE-TAPER FOR BENZODIAZEPINES, ANTI-ANXIETY, ANTICONVULSANTS AND SLEEP MEDICATION

You will begin your pre-taper by taking Body Calm, Body Calm Supreme, Beta 1, 3-D Glucan and the Essential Protein Formula. These four supplements should take care of most or all daytime anxiety, panic attacks and sleep problems. Remember, as soon as you start the pre-taper, you simultaneously begin keeping your Daily Journal.

- *Make sure to note when existing side effects stop or when there is a major improvement. This is very important.*

You will then know which supplement turns off which side effect(s) or caused the major improvement. You will need to know this to successfully complete both the pre-taper and the full taper. The pre-taper addresses the normal cycle of anxiety/insomnia/anxiety that medication usage causes.

Anxiety both first thing in the morning and again in the afternoon are *very* common side effects of benzodiazepines, anti-anxiety, anticonvulsant and sleep medications. When using these medications, by the time you are ready to go to sleep at night you are too stressed out and fatigued from dealing with anxiety difficulties all day long. Sleep simply may not happen, and you could easily end up feeling depressed due to this continuing cycle of anxiety, no sleep, anxiety, no sleep – endlessly.

If also experiencing some degree of depression, do not be surprised if the depression goes away during the pre-taper as your ability to sleep improves or the daytime anxiety abates. But, even as you start to experience relief from your symptoms, *do not change anything*; just continue with the program. There are still many, many gains available as you move through and complete The Road Back Tapering Program.

As mentioned in the chapter, General Pre-Tapering and Tapering Instructions, new supplements for the pre-taper have been added to this third edition of the book. The new supplements are:

1. Beta 1, 3-D Glucan
2. RenewPro
3. Nature's Vitamin C

4. Probiotic Supreme

Including the Beta 1, 3, D Glucan, Nature's Vitamin C and Probiotic Supreme is strongly urged. The RenewPro has replaced the Power Barley Formula and is part of both the pre-taper and taper programs and is vital.

The Probiotic Supreme can be used for sixty days and then discontinued if you wish. We have not included the Probiotic Supreme in the steps below to keep the daily schedule easier to follow. You can take 2 capsules of the Probiotic Supreme any time during the day with food. If you use birth control pills or have taken an antibiotic in the past, we urge you to use the Probiotic Supreme for sixty days.

Step 1
Goal:

- Improved sleep.
- Vast reduction or elimination of anxiety.
- Lessening or elimination of other medication-induced side effects.

Supplements you will take:

- Essential Protein Formula.
- Body Calm.
- Body Calm Supreme.
- Beta 1, 3-D Glucan

Day One:
Action:

- Rate your daytime anxiety, panic attacks, insomnia and other side effects using your Daily Journal. Rate the anxiety, sleep and any additional symptoms from 1 to 10 – number 1 being worst and number 10 no side effect or symptom remaining.

Take:

Essential Protein Formula: 1 teaspoon mixed in a liquid of your choice.

Body Calm Supreme capsule: 1 capsule.

Time: At bedtime.

Days Two, Three, Four:

Action:

- Rate your daytime anxiety, panic attacks, insomnia and other side effects using your Daily Journal. Rate the anxiety, sleep and any additional symptoms you may be experiencing from 1 to 10 – with number 1 being worst and number 10 being no side effect or symptom remaining.

- Rate the previous night's sleep first thing in the morning.

- Rate the daytime anxiety just before bedtime of that day.

Take:

Essential Protein Formula: 1 teaspoon mixed in a liquid of your choice.

Body Calm Supreme capsule: 1 capsule.

Time: First thing in the morning when you awaken.

Take: Beta 1, 3-D Glucan. 2 capsules, 100 mg each.

Time: Any time in the morning. Use only enough liquid to wash down capsules and do not have any further liquid or food until half an hour later. Ideally you would not have food half an hour before taking the Beta 1, 3-D Glucan.

The rest of the day and up until bedtime you will be alternating the Body Calm Supreme and the Body Calm every 4 hours.

> **Example:** You wake at 7 am. Start the day by taking 1 capsule of Body Calm Supreme and 1 teaspoon of Essential Protein Formula.
>
> At 11 am, take 1 Body Calm capsule and 1 teaspoon of Essential Protein Formula.
>
> At 3 pm, take 1 Body Calm Supreme capsule and 1 teaspoon of Essential Protein Formula.
>
> At 7 pm, take 1 Body Calm capsule and 1 teaspoon of Essential Protein Formula.
>
> At bedtime or 11 pm, take 1 Body Calm Supreme capsule and 1 teaspoon of Essential Protein Formula.

Action:

- **The morning of Day 5** – Rate your sleep from the night before and look over your Daily Journal regarding daytime anxiety. If you now rate your daytime anxiety at a 7 or higher and your sleep at a 7 or higher, proceed to **Step 2**.

If you do not rate yourself at a 7 or higher for daytime anxiety and sleep, continue Step 1.

Continue Step 1

In this stage, you will be adjusting the times you take each supplement and/or the quantity of each supplement used during the day or at bedtime.

Determine the scenario that fits your circumstance:

Daytime Anxiety Below a 7 Rating and Sleep at a 7 or Higher –

If your sleep was below a rating of 7 and is now at 7 or higher, you are responding very well to the Body Calm Supreme.

a. Replace the Body Calm during the daytime with the Body Calm Supreme. Take 1 capsule of Body Calm Supreme every 4 hours during the daytime and continue taking the 1 teaspoon of Essential Protein Formula at the same time as the Body Calm Supreme during the day.

Rate your daytime anxiety at the end of every day before bedtime and rate your sleep first thing in the morning and post in your Daily Journal.

Follow Step a. for 3 days.

The goal is three consecutive days with anxiety and sleep at a rating of 7 or higher. **As soon as you have 3 consecutive days at a 7 or higher, move to Step 2.**

If you improve to a 7 rating at any time DO NOT CHANGE WHAT YOU ARE DOING.

Example: You are on day number 2 of Step a. and you now rate yourself at a 7 with anxiety and sleep. Do not change anything you are doing but continue for 2additional days and see if this new trend holds. This would give you 3 full days at a 7 rating or higher.

For the rest of the pre-taper and taper process ensure you continue taking each supplement at the same time each day and night established during this step.

If this new trend of a 7 or higher rating for daytime anxiety holds for three consecutive days, proceed to Step 2.

If you are not at a 7 or higher after 8 full days following Step a. Use the following sequence:

a. Continue with the 1 Body Calm Supreme every four hours, but increase the Essential Protein Formula to 4 teaspoons with each serving.

b. Increase the Beta 1, 3-D Glucan to 2 capsules in the morning, 2 additional capsules in the early afternoon and 2 more capsules in the late afternoon. Make sure you do not consume liquid or food for half an hour after taking the Beta 1, 3-D Glucan and ideally no food half an hour before.

Rate yourself each night for the anxiety level of that day. If you feel an improvement, but not to a rating of a 7, continue with this step for 3 full days.

If no change or you are still not up to a 7 rating after 2 full days, do the following:

- **Decrease the Essential Protein Formula back down to 1 teaspoon every four hours.**

- **Keep taking the Beta 1, 3-D Glucan three times each day.**

- **Increase the Body Calm Supreme to 1 capsule every 3 hours.**

Continue this for 3 full days. Make sure to rate your daytime anxiety each night before bedtime. If on day two or three of this procedure, you now rate yourself at a 7 or higher, continue taking the supplements exactly as you have been in this stage until you have 3 consecutive days of a rating of 7 or higher with daytime anxiety and then move to Step 2.

If the daytime anxiety is still not rated at a 7 or higher, do not get discouraged, there are still options for you.

The Anxiety Reduction Chart located in the chapter "General Pre-Tapering and Tapering Instructions" shows how anxiety tends to drop as time passes when using the correct supplement. Give yourself some time.

PRE-TAPER FOR BENZODIAZEPINES, ANTI-ANXIETY,
ANTICONVULSANTS AND SLEEP MEDICATION

Other Options

There are other options available with using the Body Calm, Body Calm Liquid and the Body Calm Supreme. The next section provides further ways an individual may use, change or alter these products for anxiety and/or insomnia relief.

Body Calm capsules – You can add 1 Body Calm capsule with each Body Calm Supreme if needed. You may take as many as 3 Body Calm capsules at bedtime for sleep. You may take 1 Body Calm Supreme, along with the Body Calm at bedtime if needed.

Body Calm liquid – For some, but very few, the Body Calm liquid is the answer for daytime anxiety and/or insomnia. Making the switch from capsule to liquid can be magic.

Body Calm Supreme – As described in the chapter "General Pre-Tapering and Tapering Instructions," reaching a "steady state" can be different for each person. If you are feeling some relief from anxiety, but only temporarily, you may need to change the frequency or amount of Body Calm Supreme. You can take the Body Calm Supreme every 2 hours during the day to achieve this. This gives astounding results for some people.

As mentioned earlier in this chapter you can take the Nature's Vitamin C and Probiotic Supreme. If the adrenals need help introduce the Nature's Vitamin C. The adrenals require ample supply of vitamin C to work properly.

Most medications create a yeast overgrowth which the Probiotic Supreme handles quickly. Side effects from yeast overgrowth can include anxiety, depression and insomnia.

Daytime anxiety – Daytime anxiety may also be helped by including CLA daily. You would take 1 softgel in the morning, again at noon and once more before 4 pm. Make sure to include 1 Ultimate Omega 3 in the morning and at noon along with one vitamin E in the morning.

We have tried to remove all trial and success out of this program but sometimes there are no other options. The Nature's Vitamin C, Probiotic

Supreme and CLA are trial and success. They may not make a change or they may be the exact fit for your body. Use these at this stage to see if they are what your body needs to get over this hump.

Suggestions: If you have felt any improvement during these procedures, you have something to work with. If the anxiety has at least moved from a rating of 3 to a 5, and is holding at that level, using these supplements will be the answer to your success. You will need to adjust them further, allow a little additional time, or adjust the time of day you are taking them. Adjust supplements one-by-one every third day. Keep good notes in your journal. The answers vary between the quantity and how often a supplement is taken. The answer can also be both quantity and frequency of taking the supplement.

Experiment with these variables as needed and keep your Daily Journal. Allow some time for results. If you have had some improvement, such as from a 3 to a 5 rating, and it is holding steady, but will not move beyond a 5 rating, give this stage 30 days to fully work.

After 30 days, if still at a 5 rating, move on to Step 2 and keep rating the daytime anxiety each evening. It may very well improve to a 7 rating later in the pre-taper.

A blood test can verify the level of a substance called Interleukin-2 (IL-2). The reference range for IL-2 will be from 223 to 710 with most laboratories. If your test results come back with a level under 466, you need to increase the IL-2 further and should increase the Beta 1, 3-D Glucan to a total of 9 capsules each day.

Increase the Beta 1, 3-D Glucan to 3 of the 100 mg capsules 3 times a day. Give this increase 14 days to completely work. If you have improved after 14 days but are not up to a 7 rating yet, you can increase the Beta 1, 3-D Glucan to 2,500 mg each day if needed. Increase by no more than 300 mg every 3 days.

PRE-TAPER FOR BENZODIAZEPINES, ANTI-ANXIETY, ANTICONVULSANTS AND SLEEP MEDICATION

Daytime Anxiety Above a 7 Rating and Sleep Below a 7 Rating -

a. Keep doing exactly what you have been doing during the daytime, during Step 1.

b. Keep in mind as you increase the supplements for sleep that changes made during the daytime for the anxiety may very well help with sleep as well. If a person who previously had daytime anxiety no longer has such, the chances are very high that their ability to sleep will improve greatly.

Do: Increase the Body Calm Supreme to 2 capsules at bedtime and continue to take the 1 teaspoon of Essential Protein Formula. Take 2 additional 100 mg capsules of Beta 1, 3-D Glucan after 4 pm but before 8 pm.

Stay at this level for 3 nights.

Make sure to rate your night's sleep each morning upon waking.

If you rate yourself at a 7 or higher on any of these 3 nights, continue with exactly what you are doing until you have 3 consecutive nights of sleep rated at 7 or higher. Then move to Step 2.

If sleep drops below a 7 after being at a 7 or higher for one or two days but not the 3 consecutive days, increase the Essential Protein Formula to 4 teaspoons at bedtime and continue taking the 2 Body Calm Supreme capsules at bedtime as well. Continue with the Beta 1, 3-D Glucan as well.

See if this gives you the 3 consecutive nights of sleep at a 7 rating or higher and then move to Step 2. If it does not, reduce the Essential Protein Formula back to a 1 teaspoon serving.

c. If b. did not result in the desired rating of a 7 or higher, include 1 Body Calm capsule at bedtime, along with the 2 Body Calm Supreme capsules, and the 1 teaspoon of Essential Protein Formula. Continue with the additional Beta 1, 3-D Glucan.

If there is no change in 3 nights, increase the Body Calm capsules to 2 at bedtime, along with the 2 Body Calm Supreme capsules and the 1 teaspoon of Essential Protein Formula. Continue with the additional Beta 1, 3-D Glucan.

Again, wait 3 days and see if sleep improves to a 7 or higher. Then move to Step 2 after 3 consecutive days of this 7 or higher rating.

d. If you are having difficulty going to sleep, try taking all the supplements half an hour before bedtime for 3 nights. If still no change, try taking the supplements 1 hour before bedtime for 3 nights. If you begin to feel tired before your normal bedtime, go to bed a little earlier than usual. This may be your window of opportunity to fall asleep with ease; you do not want to miss that chance.

e. If you are waking up in the middle of the night and are able to go back to sleep with little effort, that is normal. If you have difficulty going back to sleep, take 1 Body Calm Supreme in the night when you waken.

f. If at any time you begin to sleep well with a 7 or higher rating, but you wake up tired, reduce the last supplement that was increased slightly. You can open up any of the capsules and remove half of the supplement powder.

Reaching Stage 2 of deeper sleep requires IL-2. If IL-2 levels are too low you will have difficulty going into deep restful sleep. You can increase the Beta 1, 3-D Glucan to 3 of the 100 mg capsules 3 times a day. Allow 14 days for this increase to work. If you feel improvement after 14 days but are not yet up to a 7 rating, you can increase the Beta 1, 3-D Glucan to 2,500 mg each day if needed. Increase by no more than 300 mg every 3 days.

PRE-TAPER FOR BENZODIAZEPINES, ANTI-ANXIETY, ANTICONVULSANTS AND SLEEP MEDICATION

Remember, **have 3 consecutive nights at a 7 rating or higher for sleep and then move to Step 2**.

Suggestions: If you have felt any improvement during this procedure, you have something to work with. If the insomnia has at least moved from a 3 to a 5 rating, and is holding at that level, these supplements will be the answer to your success. You just need to adjust them further, allow a little additional time or adjust the time of day you are taking them. Adjust supplements one-by-one every third day. Keep good notes in your journal. The answer will either be the quantity of a supplement or how often the supplement is taken.

Experiment with this and keep your Daily Journal. Give this some time to work. If you have had some improvement, such as from a 3 to a 5 rating, and it is holding steady, but will not move beyond a 5 rating, give this stage 30 days to fully work.

After 30 days, if still at a 5 rating, move on to Step 2 and keep rating your sleep each evening. It may very well improve to a 7 rating later in the pre-taper.

Special Note: If taking calcium and still not at a 7 rating or higher, you need to remove the calcium supplement or at least add Calsorption and see if the additional calcium absorption helps. If taking other supplements not part of The Road Back Program, it is time for you to quit taking them.

If your healthcare provider suggested other supplements, let the practitioner know what you want to do, and give the practitioner this book. Once you are off all other supplements for 3 full days, you should feel a remarkable difference.

Daytime Anxiety Below a 7 Rating and Sleep Below a 7 Rating

a. Increase Body Calm Supreme to 1 capsule every 2 hours during the day.

b. Take 1 teaspoon of Essential Protein Formula with every Body Calm Supreme.

c. Take Probiotic Supreme as directed on the bottle each day.

d. Take 3 capsules of Nature's Vitamin C each day. Take 1 in the morning, one at noon and one additional capsule before 4 pm.

e. Take 1 softgel of CLA in the morning, 1 softgel at noon and 1 softgel at 4 pm.

f. Take 1 softgel of Ultimate Omega 3 in the morning, 1 at noon and 1 more softgel at 4 pm.

g. Take 1 softgel of vitamin E in the morning.

If you have read further in this chapter you will notice you are doing part of Step 2 of the pre-taper. Once you have your anxiety and sleep rating at a 7 or above in this step and that rating has held for 3 consecutive days, you are ready to move to Step 3 of the pre-taper.

Make sure to keep your Daily Journal as well as your daily graphs for your 1-10 rating. Note all changes made in supplements and when made. When a positive change happens it is usually from some change that took place in the past 3 days.

If you do not rate yourself at a 7 or higher after 7 full days using this approach move to Step 3. Step 3 may be the supplement that gets you over the top.

If you complete all stages for anxiety and sleep and you still rate anxiety and sleep below a 7 on a 1-10 scale, one of these nine things are probably happening:

PRE-TAPER FOR BENZODIAZEPINES, ANTI-ANXIETY, ANTICONVULSANTS AND SLEEP MEDICATION

1. You are one of the few who need to continue taking the supplements for additional time before they will work for you.

   This happens rarely.

2. You need to reevaluate how you are rating yourself. Are you being a little too rough on how you are judging yourself?

   Reread the section in the chapter, "General Pre-Tapering and Tapering Instructions."

   Keep in mind, if you had anxiety throughout the day which was extreme, and the anxiety now occurs only in the morning when you wake up then disappears for the rest of the day, you have had a major positive change.

   Review all the sleep scenarios in the chapter, "General Pre-Tapering and Tapering Instructions." Before starting Step 1 of the Pre-Taper, if you previously woke up in the middle of the night and had a difficult time going back to sleep, but now wake up in the middle of the night and instantly go back to sleep, this is a major positive change.

3. You are taking other supplements and the reason you are unresponsive to Stage 1 is those supplements. This is where you need to reevaluate calcium (if you are taking it), B vitamins and all other supplements. The other supplements, herbs or concoctions may have been causing the increased anxiety or insomnia for some time.

   These other supplements might be excellent, but not when you are taking these types of medications.

   Meet with your doctor. Ask him or her if you can quit taking other supplements that are not part of The Road Back Program. If OK with your doctor, discontinue the other supplements. Continue taking the supplements used during Step 1 of the Pre-Taper. Give yourself 3 days and see how you are doing.

4. You are changing something.

5. You are not taking the supplements as outlined.

6. Maybe you are changing the time of day when you take your medication.

7. Look at the weekends. Are you sleeping in a few hours later and not taking the morning medication at the same time? Are you staying up later in the evening thus not taking the medication at the same time each day?

   Have you changed anything in your daily routine?

8. You started The Road Back Program after you had already made one or several attempts to come off your medication and were having withdrawal side effects before starting the program.

   You should give Step 1 additional time. Many people respond quickly to this step, even if they fit into this category, but some require from 14 to 30 days to fully complete Step 1 when they fit in this group.

   Give it some time, at least the 30 days.

9. The Road Back Program is not for you. I wish I could say this program works for everyone, but it does not. From years of experience, I know the program does not work for a very low percentage of people, but there is that percentage nonetheless.

   You have not caused additional harm by your attempt.

Step 2

- Continue taking all supplements as established during Step 1.

Goal:

- Improvement of Mood.

- A lessening or elimination of other medication-induced side effects.

Supplement you will introduce:

- Ultimate Omega 3.

Day One:

Action:

- Rate your mood and other side effects. Use the Daily Journal and rate your mood and any additional symptoms you may be experiencing from 1 to 10. Rate with number 1 being the worst and number 10 being no side effect or symptom remaining. Keep rating the anxiety and sleep as you were during Step 1.

Take: 1 softgel of Ultimate Omega 3.

Time: First thing in the morning, and around noon, but before 4 pm.

Day Two, Three, Four:

Action:

- Rate your mood and other side effects. Use the Daily Journal and rate your mood and any additional symptoms you may be experiencing from 1 to 10. Rate with number 1 being the worst and number 10 being no side effect or symptom remaining.

Take: 2 Ultimate Omega 3 softgels.

Time: First thing in the morning when you awaken, and around noon, but before 4 pm.

After the rigors of Step 1, you will find Step 2 to be quick and easy. You are finished and ready to move to Step 3.

Step 3

- Continue taking all supplements as established during Steps 1 and 2.

Goal:

- Overall brightness of feelings and mood.
- Nice and smooth energy level.
- A lessening or elimination of other medication induced side effects.

Supplement you will introduce:

- RenewPro.

Day One:

Action:

- Rate anxiety, sleep and all side effects. Use the Daily Journal and rate your mood, anxiety sleep, and any additional symptoms you may be experiencing, from 1 to 10. Rate with number 1 being the worst and number 10 being no side effect or symptom remaining.

Take: 1/2 scoop of RenewPro.

Time: First thing in the morning.

Day Two, Three, Four:

Action:

- Rate anxiety, sleep and all side effects. Use the Daily Journal and rate your mood, anxiety, sleep and any additional symptoms you may be experiencing, from 1 to 10. Rate with number 1 being the worst and number 10 being no side effect or symptom remaining.

Take: 1/2 scoop of RenewPro.

Time: First thing in the morning, around noon and one more before 4 pm.

Step 4

Day 1:

Begin taking 400 i.u. of vitamin E first thing in the morning with the rest of the morning supplements.

Keep taking all supplements exactly as you have established during the pre-taper while you taper off the medication and continue for 45 days after the last dosage of the medication.

You are completely finished with the pre-taper when:

- You rate yourself at a 7 or higher for anxiety and sleep.

The supplements and how much you take of each supplement may be changed during the taper portion of the program. Follow the exact instructions outlined in the taper chapter you are going to follow.

If you have tried to quit these medications in the past, you may be a little apprehensive about reducing them again. You can remain at this stage of the process for as long as you like. You do not have to rush.

It is now time to decide which taper program to follow. You can now taper off the medication twice as fast with this program if desired. The slower method has been kept in the book if you wish to really take your time with the taper portion.

The two chapters are:

- How to Taper Off Benzodiazepines, Anti-anxiety, Anticonvulsant and Sleep Medication. *The Slow and Gradual Taper.*

- How to Taper Off Benzodiazepines, Anti-anxiety, Anticonvulsant, and Sleep Medication. *The Fast and Gradual Taper.*

CHAPTER 10

PRE-TAPER FOR CYMBALTA

"Your program is the best thing I have done for myself in a very long time. I have been taking an anti-depressant of one type or another for the past 16 years. I have tried to taper off of them before, but with no luck. I started to accept the fact that I would be taking this for the rest of my life. Then I found "The Road Back." I am almost done tapering completely off of the meds and what withdrawals I have felt I have been able to alleviate them almost immediately by adjusting the supplements. Thank you, Thank you, Thank you!"

Linda M.

If you have not read the entire chapter "General Pre-Tapering and Tapering Instructions," please do so before continuing with this chapter. Reading and understanding the chapter "General Pre-Tapering and Tapering Instructions" is vital before starting the pre-taper.

Starting Your Pre-Taper

The pre-taper for Cymbalta is divided into two separate pre-taper programs to accommodate the side effects you currently experience.

If you are suffering from anxiety and insomnia, use the Anxiety Insomnia Pre-taper.

If you do not have anxiety and insomnia, use the Fatigue Pre-taper.

As mentioned in the chapter, *General Pre-Tapering and Tapering Instructions*, new supplements have been added to this third edition of the book for this pre-taper.

The new supplements for this pre-taper and taper are:

1. Beta 1, 3-D Glucan
2. RenewPro
3. Nature's Vitamin C
4. Probiotic Supreme

It is strongly urged you include the Beta 1, 3, D Glucan, Nature's Vitamin C and the Probiotic Supreme. The RenewPro has replaced the Power Barley Formula if you have anxiety or insomnia and is part of this pre-taper and taper program and needs to be used.

The Probiotic Supreme can be used for 60 days then discontinued if you wish. I have not included the Probiotic Supreme in the steps below in an attempt to keep the daily schedule easier to follow. You can take 2 capsules of the Probiotic Supreme any time during the day with food. If you use birth control pills or have taken an antibiotic in the past, you should use the Probiotic Supreme for the 60 days. Clinical trials have shown at least 18% of all people that use or have used an antidepressant will have Candida yeast overgrowth. With side effects associated with Candida yeast overgrowth, you should use this probiotic.

PRE-TAPER PROGRAM
IF YOU HAVE DAYTIME ANXIETY,
AGITATION OR INSOMNIA OR ARE
TAKING AN ANTIPSYCHOTIC

As you are experiencing chronic anxiety during the day and insomnia at night as side effects of Cymbalta, you will start your pre-taper with Body Calm, Body Calm Supreme, Beta 1, 3-D Glucan and Essential Protein Formula; products specifically formulated to help relieve these symptoms.

With either anxiety or insomnia present, there are sure to be other symptoms as well, most likely caused by your anxiety during the day and lack of sleep at night.

You will begin your pre-taper by taking Body Calm, Body Calm Supreme, Beta 1, 3-D Glucan and the Essential Protein Formula as directed in this chapter. These four supplements should take care of all or most of the daytime anxiety, panic attacks and sleep problems. Remember, as soon as you start the pre-taper, you will simultaneously start keeping track of your days in the Daily Journal.

Make sure to note when existing side effects stop or when there is a major improvement. This is very important.

You will then know which supplement turns off which side effect(s) or caused the major improvement. You will need to know this in order to complete both the pre-taper and the full taper successfully. The pre-taper is designed to address the normal cycle of anxiety/insomnia/anxiety that takes place because of Cymbalta.

Anxiety first thing in the morning and a return of the anxiety in the afternoon are both *very* common side effects.

On any given day when using Cymbalta, by the time you are ready to go to sleep at night you are too stressed out and fatigued from dealing with the difficulties of the anxiety all day long. Sleep simply may not happen, and you could easily end up feeling depressed due to this continuing cycle of anxiety, no sleep, anxiety, no sleep, endlessly.

If you are also experiencing some degree of depression, do not be surprised if it goes away during the pre-taper, as your ability to sleep improves or the daytime anxiety abates. But, as you start to experience relief from your symptoms, *do not change anything*; just continue with the program. There are still many, many gains to be had as you move through to full completion of The Road Back Tapering Program.

Step 1

Goal:

- Improved sleep.
- A vast reduction or elimination of anxiety.
- A lessening or elimination of other Cymbalta-induced side effects.

Supplements you will take:

- Essential Protein Formula.
- Body Calm.
- Body Calm Supreme.
- Beta 1, 3-D Glucan.

Day One:

Action:

- Rate your daytime anxiety, panic attacks, insomnia and other side effects. Use the Daily Journal and rate anxiety, sleep and any additional symptoms you may be experiencing from 1 to 10. Rate with number 1 being the worst and number 10 being no side effect or symptom remaining.

Take: Essential Protein Formula: 1 teaspoon mixed in a liquid of your choice.

Body Calm Supreme capsule: 1 capsule.

Time: At bedtime.

Day Two, Three, Four:

Action:

- Rate your daytime anxiety, panic attacks, insomnia and other side effects. Use the Daily Journal and rate anxiety, sleep and any additional symptoms you may be experiencing from 1 to 10. Rate with number 1 being the worst and number 10 being no side effect or symptom remaining.
- Rate the previous night's sleep first thing the next morning.
- Rate the daytime anxiety just before bedtime of that day.

Take: Essential Protein Formula: 1 teaspoon mixed in a liquid of your choice.

Body Calm Supreme capsule: 1 capsule.

Time: First thing in the morning when you awaken.

Take: Beta 1, 3-D Glucan. Take 1 capsule of 100 mg Beta 1, 3-D Glucan.

Time: Any time in the morning. Make sure to only use as much liquid as needed to wash the capsule down and drink no other liquid or food for half an hour after taking the supplement. Ideally, you would not have food half an hour before taking the Beta 1, 3-D Glucan.

The rest of the day and up until bedtime, you will be alternating the Body Calm Supreme and the Body Calm every 4 hours.

Example: You wake up at 7 am. You would start the day by taking 1 capsule of Body Calm Supreme and 1 teaspoon of Essential Protein Formula.

At 11 am, you would take 1 Body Calm capsule and 1 teaspoon of Essential Protein Formula.

At 3 pm, you would take 1 Body Calm Supreme capsule and 1 teaspoon of Essential Protein Formula.

At 7 pm, you would take 1 Body Calm capsule and 1 teaspoon of Essential Protein Formula.

At bedtime, or 11 pm, you would take 1 Body Calm Supreme capsule and 1 teaspoon of Essential Protein Formula.

Action:

- **The morning of Day 5** – Rate your sleep from the night before and have a look at your Daily Journal regarding daytime anxiety. If you now rate your daytime anxiety at a 7 or higher and your sleep is at a 7 or higher, proceed to **Step 2**.

If you do not rate yourself at a 7 or higher for daytime anxiety and sleep, continue Step 1.

Continue Step 1

In this stage, you will be adjusting the time you take each supplement and/or the quantity of each supplement used during the day or at bedtime.

Locate the scenario that fits your circumstance:

Daytime Anxiety Below a 7 Rating and Sleep at a 7 0r Higher

If your sleep was below a rating of a 7 and is now at a 7 or higher, you are responding very well to the Body Calm Supreme.

a. Replace the Body Calm during the daytime with the Body Calm Supreme. Take 1 capsule of Body Calm Supreme every 4 hours during the daytime and continue taking the 1 teaspoon of Essential Protein Formula at the same time as the Body Calm Supreme during the day.

Rate your daytime anxiety at the end of every day before bedtime and rate your sleep first thing in the morning and post in your Daily Journal.

Follow Step a. for 3 days.

The goal is to have three consecutive days with anxiety and sleep at a rating of 7 or higher. **As soon as you have 3 consecutive days at a 7 or higher, move to Step 2.**

If you improve to a 7 rating at any time, **DO NOT CHANGE WHAT YOU ARE DOING.**

Example: You are on day number 2 of Step a. and you now rate yourself at a 7 with anxiety and sleep. Do not change anything you are doing, but continue for 2 additional days and see if this new trend holds. This would give you 3 full days at a 7 rating or higher.

Make sure to continue taking each supplement at the same times that you've established during this step for the rest of the pre-taper and taper process.

If this new trend of a 7 or higher rating for daytime anxiety holds for three consecutive days, proceed to Step 2.

If you are not at a 7 or higher after 8 full days, following Step a., use the following sequence:

Continue with the 1 Body Calm Supreme every four hours but increase the Essential Protein Formula to 4 teaspoons with each serving.

Rate yourself each night for the anxiety level of that day. If you feel an improvement, but not to a rating of a 7, continue with this step for 2 full days. If there is no change, or you are still not up to a 7 rating after 2 full days, do the following:

Decrease the Essential Protein Formula back down to 1 teaspoon every four hours.

Begin taking 6 Beta 1, 3-D Glucan daily. Take 2 in the morning, 2 additional capsules near noon and 2 more capsules before 4 pm.

Increase the Body Calm Supreme to 1 capsule every 3 hours.

Continue this for 3 full days. Make sure to rate your daytime anxiety each night before bedtime. If on day two or three of this procedure you now rate yourself at a 7 or higher, continue taking the supplements exactly as you have been in this stage until you have 3 consecutive days of a rating of 7 or higher with daytime anxiety, and then move to Step 2.

If your daytime anxiety is still not rated at a 7 or higher, do not get discouraged, there are still options for you.

The Anxiety Reduction Chart located in the chapter "General Pre-Tapering and Tapering Instructions," shows how anxiety tends to drop as time passes when using the correct supplement. Give this some time.

Other Options

There are other options available with using the Body Calm, Body Calm Liquid and the Body Calm Supreme. The next section provides further ways you may change or alter this routine for anxiety and or insomnia.

Body Calm capsules – You can add 1 Body Calm capsule with each Body Calm Supreme if needed. You can take as many as 3 Body Calm capsules at bedtime for sleep.

Body Calm liquid – For very few, the Body Calm liquid is the answer for daytime anxiety and or insomnia. Switching from capsule to liquid can be magic.

Body Calm Supreme – As described in the chapter "General Pre-Tapering and Tapering Instructions," reaching a "steady state" can be different for each person. If you are feeling some relief from anxiety, but it is only temporary, you may need to change the frequency or amount of Body Calm Supreme. You can take the Body Calm Supreme every 2 hours during the day to achieve this. For some people this makes astounding results.

Suggestions: If you have felt any improvement during these procedures, you have something to work with. If the anxiety has at least moved from a 3 to a 5 rating, and the anxiety is holding at that level, using these supplements will be the answer for your success. You just need to adjust them further, allow a little additional time, or adjust the time of day you are taking them. Adjust supplements one-by-one every third day. Keep good notes in your journal. The answers will be either the quantity taken of a supplement or how often the supplement is taken. However, the answer can be both quantity and how often a supplement is taken.

Experiment with this as needed and keep your Daily Journal. Give this some time to work. If you have had some improvement, such as from a 3 to a 5 rating, and it is holding steady, but will not move beyond a 5 rating, give this stage 30-days to fully work.

After 30-days, if still at a 5 rating, move on to Step 2 and keep rating the daytime anxiety each evening. It may very well improve to a 7 rating later in the pre-taper.

Daytime Anxiety Above a 7 Rating and Sleep Below a 7 Rating

    a. Keep doing exactly what you have been doing during the daytime during

Step 1.

    b. One thing here to keep in mind as you increase the supplements for sleep, the changes made during the daytime for the anxiety may very well help with the sleep, as well. If a person who had daytime anxiety no longer has daytime anxiety, the chances are very high that his or her ability to sleep will improve greatly as well.

Do: Increase the Body Calm Supreme to 2 capsules at bedtime and continue to take the 1-teaspoon of Essential Protein Formula.

Stay at this level for 3 nights.

Make sure to rate your sleep each morning when you awake for the night before.

If you rate yourself at a 7 or higher any of these 3 nights, continue with exactly what you are doing until you have 3 consecutive nights of a sleep rated at 7 or higher. Then move to Step 2.

If sleep drops below a 7 after being at a 7 or higher for one or two days, but not the 3 consecutive days, increase the Essential Protein Formula to 4 teaspoons at bedtime and continue taking the 2 Body Calm Supreme capsules at bedtime as well.

See if this will get you the 3 consecutive nights of sleep at a 7 rating or higher and then move to Step 2. If it does not, reduce the Essential Protein Formula back to a 1 teaspoon serving.

c. If b. did not result in the desired rating of a 7 or higher, include 1 Body Calm capsule at bedtime, along with the 2 Body Calm Supreme capsules and the 1 teaspoon of Essential Protein Formula.

If there is no change in 3 nights, increase the Body Calm capsules to 2 at bedtime along with the 2 Body Calm Supreme capsules and the 1 teaspoon of Essential Protein Formula.

Again, wait 3 days and see if sleep improves to a 7 or higher, and then move to Step 2 after 3 consecutive days of this 7 or higher rating.

d. If you are having difficulty going to sleep, try taking all the supplements ½ hour before bedtime for 3 nights. If still no change, try taking the supplements 1 hour before bedtime for 3 nights. If you begin to feel tired before your normal bedtime, go to bed a little earlier than usual. This may be your window of opportunity for going to sleep with ease, and we do not want to miss the chance.

e. If you are waking up in the middle of the night and are able to go back to sleep with little effort, that is very normal. If you have difficulty going back to sleep, take 1 Body Calm Supreme in the night when you awaken.

f. If at any time you begin to sleep well with a 7 or higher rating, but you wake up tired, reduce the last supplement that was increased slightly. You can open up any of the capsules and remove ½ of the supplement powder.

***Remember*, have 3 consecutive nights at a 7 rating or higher for sleep and then move to Step 2**.

Body Calm capsules – There have been a few people that needed to take 3 Body Calm capsules at bedtime, along with the other supplements to reach a good night sleep at a 7 or higher rating.

Body Calm liquid – For some but very few, the Body Calm liquid was the answer for sleep. Making the switch from capsule to liquid can be magic.

Body Calm Supreme – As described in the chapter *General Pre-Tapering and Tapering Instructions,* reaching a "steady state" can be different for each person. If you are feeling some relief from insomnia but it is not enough, you may need to change the amount of Body Calm Supreme. It may take 3 Body Calm Supreme capsules to fully handle the insomnia.

Suggestions: If you have felt any improvement during these procedures, you have something to work with. If the insomnia has at least moved from a rating of 3 to a 5 rating, and the insomnia is holding at that level, using these supplements will be the answer for your success. You just need to adjust them further, allow a little additional time, or adjust the time of day you are taking them. Adjust supplements one-by-one every third day. Keep good notes in your journal. The answers will either be the quantity of a supplement taken or how often. However, the answer can be both quantity and how often a supplement is taken.

Experiment with these and keep your Daily Journal. Give this some time to work. If you have had some improvement, such as from a 3 to a 5 rating, and it is holding steady but will not move beyond a 5 rating, give this stage 30 days to fully work.

After 30 days, if still at a 5 rating, move on to Step 2 and keep rating your sleep each evening. It may very well improve to a 7 rating later in the pre-taper.

Special Note: If you have insisted on taking calcium and you still are not at a 7 rating or higher, remove the calcium supplement. If you are taking other supplements that are not part of The Road Back Program, it is time for you to quit taking them.

If your healthcare provider suggested other supplements, let the practitioner know what you want to do, and take the practitioner a printout this book. Once you are off all other supplements for 3 full days, you should feel a remarkable difference.

Daytime Anxiety Below a 7 Rating and Sleep Below a 7 Rating.

If you complete all stages for anxiety and sleep and still rate anxiety and sleep below a 7 on a 1-10 scale, one of these nine things is happening:

1. You are one of the few who need to continue taking the supplements for additional time before they will work for you.

   This happens rarely.

2. You need to reevaluate how you are rating yourself. Are you being a little too rough on how you are judging yourself?

   Reread the section in the chapter, "General Pre-Tapering and Tapering Instructions."

   Keep in mind, if you had anxiety throughout the day which was extreme, and the anxiety is now only in the morning when you wake up, and then disappears for the rest of the day, you have had a major positive change.

   Review all the sleep scenarios in the chapter, "General Pre-Tapering and Tapering Instructions." Before starting Step 1 of the Pre-Taper, if you used to wake up in the middle of the night and had a difficult time going back to sleep, but now you wake up in the middle of the night and instantly go back to sleep, this is a major positive change.

3. You are taking other supplements and the real reason you will not respond to Stage 1 is the other supplements. This is when you need to reevaluate calcium (if you are taking it), B vitamins and all other supplements. The other supplements, herbs or concoctions may have been causing the increased anxiety or insomnia for some time.

These other supplements might be excellent but not when you are taking medication from this group.

See your doctor. Ask your doctor if you can quit taking the other supplements that are not part of The Road Back Program. If OK with your doctor, discontinue the other supplements. Continue taking the supplements used during Step 1 of the Pre-Taper. Give yourself 3 days and see how you are doing.

4. You are changing something.
5. You are not taking the supplements as outlined.
6. Maybe you are changing the time of day when you take your medication.
7. Look at the weekends. Are you sleeping in a few hours later and not taking the morning medication at the same time? Are you staying up later in the evening thus not taking the medication at the same time?

Have you changed anything in your daily routine?

8. You have started The Road Back Program after you have already made one or several attempts to come off your medication and were having withdrawal side effects before starting the program.

You should give Step 1 additional time. Many people respond quickly to this step, even if they fit into this category, but some require from 14 to 30 days to fully complete Step 1.

9. Give it some time, at least the 30 days.

The Road Back Program is not for you. I wish I could say this program works for everyone, but it does not. From many years experience, I know that this program will not work for a very small percentage of people, but there is that percentage, nonetheless.

10. You have not caused additional harm by your attempt.

Step 2

- Continue taking all supplements as established during Step 1.

Goal:

- Improvement of mood.
- A lessening or elimination of other Cymbalta induced side effects.

Supplement you will introduce:

- Ultimate Omega 3.

Day One:

Action:

- Rate your mood and other side effects. Use the Daily Journal and rate your mood and any additional symptoms you may be experiencing from 1 to 10. Rate with number 1 being the worst and number 10 being no side effect or symptoms remaining.

Take: 2 Ultimate Omega 3 softgels.

Time: First thing in the morning and around noon, but before 4 pm.

Day Two, Three, Four:

Action:

- Rate your mood and other side effects. Use the Daily Journal and rate mood and any additional symptoms you may be experiencing from 1 to 10. Rate with number 1 being the worst and number 10 being no side effect or symptom remaining.

Take: 3 Ultimate Omega 3 softgels.

Time: First thing in the morning when you awaken, and around noon, but before 4 pm.

After the rigors of Step 1, you will find Step 2 quick and easy. You are finished and ready to move to Step 3.

You are finished increasing the Ultimate Omega 3. Move to Step 3 even if there has not been a major positive change with the last increase of Omega 3.

Step 3

- Continue taking all supplements as established during Steps 1 and 2.

Goal:

- Overall brightness of feelings and mood.
- Nice and smooth energy level.
- A lessening or elimination of other medication induced side effects.

Supplement you will introduce:

- RenewPro.

Day One:

Action:

- Rate anxiety, sleep and all side effects. Use the Daily Journal and rate your mood, anxiety, sleep and any additional symptoms you may be experiencing from 1 to 10. Rate with number 1 being the worst and number 10 being no side effect or symptom remaining.

Take: 1/2 scoop of RenewPro.

Time: First thing in the morning.

Day Two, Three, Four:

Action:

- Rate anxiety, sleep and all side effects. Use the Daily Journal and rate your mood, anxiety, sleep and any additional symptoms you may be experiencing from 1 to 10. Rate with number 1 being the worst and number 10 being no side effect or symptom remaining.

Take: 1/2 scoop of RenewPro

Time: First thing in the morning and around noon.

Step 4

Day 1:

Begin taking 400 i.u. of vitamin E first thing in the morning. Take the vitamin E with the rest of the morning supplements.

Begin taking 1 capsule of Nature's Vitamin C any time around midday. **(If you are taking ADHD Medication do not take any vitamin C and watch your fruit intake.)**

Keep taking all supplements exactly as you have established during the pre-taper.

You are completely finished with the pre-taper when:

- 22 days have passed after you started Step 1

  and

- You rate yourself at a 7 or higher for anxiety and sleep.

You do need to wait the 22 days from the date you started Step 1, even if you are at a 7 rating or higher for anxiety and insomnia.

Continue taking all of the supplements exactly as you are now during the tapering portion of the medication.

If you have tried to quit these medications in the past, you may be a little apprehensive about reducing the medication again. You can remain at this stage of the process for as long as you like. You do not have to rush.

When you are ready, follow the procedures detailed in the chapter, How to Taper off Cymbalta (Slow and Gradual) or the next chapter How to Taper off Cymbalta (Fast and Gradual).

PRE-TAPER PROGRAM
IF YOU HAVE FATIGUE and DO NOT
HAVE ANXIETY OR INSOMNIA

Supplement you will introduce:

- Power Barley Formula.

- **Special Note**: You will be increasing the Power Barley Formula slowly over a number of days. The word "Power" in the name is intentional. This barley formula is powerful and unlike any other barley product.

  At any time during the pre-taper, when you feel increased energy, a new brightness about yourself, an overall good feeling, DO NOT INCREASE THE POWER BARLEY FORMULA FURTHER.

  The pre-taper schedule has you increasing the Power Barley Formula over a number of days but if taking the Power Barley Formula only once in the morning gives you an increased energy, a new brightness about yourself, an overall good feeling, do not increase it further.

  If an amount of barley that is less than 1 tablespoon brings on the positive change, keep taking that amount of barley for 7 consecutive days before moving on to Step 2.

Day One:

Action:

- Rate fatigue, anxiety, sleep and all side effects. Use the Daily Journal and rate your fatigue, mood, anxiety, sleep and other additional symptoms you may be experiencing from 1 to 10. Rate with number

1 being the worst and number 10 being no side effect or symptom remaining.

Take: 1/2 teaspoon of Power Barley Formula.

Time: First thing in the morning.

Day Two, Three, Four:

Action:

- Rate fatigue, anxiety, sleep and all side effects. Use the Daily Journal and rate your fatigue, mood, anxiety, sleep and any additional symptoms you may be experiencing from 1 to 10. Rate with number 1 being the worst and number 10 being no side effect or symptom remaining.

Take: 1/2 teaspoon of Power Barley Formula.

Time: First thing in the morning, around noon and once again before 4 pm.

* Remember, this barley formula is not like other barley products. When you feel the positive change, remain where you are, do not increase further. If you went past the positive point and you do not feel as well, return to the last amount of barley you were taking.

Day Five, Six, Seven:

Action:

- Rate fatigue, anxiety, sleep and all side effects. Use the Daily Journal and rate your fatigue, mood, anxiety, sleep and any additional symptoms you may be experiencing from 1 to 10. Rate with number 1 being the worst and number 10 being no side effect or symptom remaining.

Take: 1 teaspoon of Power Barley Formula.

Time: First thing in the morning, around noon and once again before 4 pm.

If no major positive changes, continue with Day Eight, Nine and Ten. If the major positive changes took place during this part, move to Step 2.

Day Eight, Nine, Ten:

Action:

- Rate fatigue, anxiety, sleep and all side effects. Use the Daily Journal and rate your fatigue, mood, anxiety, sleep and any additional symptoms you may be experiencing from 1 to 10. Rate with number 1 being the worst and number 10 being no side effect or symptom remaining.

Take: 2 teaspoons of Power Barley Formula.

Time: First thing in the morning, around noon and once again before 4 pm.

Day Eleven, Twelve, Thirteen:

Action:

- Rate fatigue, anxiety, sleep and all side effects. Use the Daily Journal and rate your fatigue, mood, anxiety, sleep and any additional symptoms you may be experiencing from 1 to 10. Rate with number 1 being the worst and number 10 being no side effect or symptom remaining.

Take: 1 *tablespoon* of Power Barley Formula.

Time: First thing in the morning, around noon and once again before 4 pm.

You are ready to move to Step 2.

Step 2

- **Continue taking all supplements as established during Step 1.**

Goal:

- Improvement of mood.
- A lessening or elimination of other medication induced side effects.

Supplement you will introduce:

- Ultimate Omega 3.

Day One:

Action:

- Rate your mood and other side effects. Use the Daily Journal and rate your mood and any additional symptoms you may be experiencing from 1 to 10. Rate with number 1 being the worst and number 10 being no side effect or symptom remaining.

Take: 2 Ultimate Omega 3 softgels

Time: First thing in the morning and around noon but before 4 pm.

Day Two, Three, Four:

Action:

- Rate your mood and other side effects. Use the Daily Journal and rate mood and any additional symptoms you may be experiencing from 1 to 10. Rate with number 1 being the worst and number 10 being no side effect or symptom remaining.

Take: 3 Ultimate Omega 3 softgels.

Time: First thing in the morning when you awake and around noon but before 4 pm.

Day Five, Six, Seven:

Action:

- Rate your mood and other side effects. Use the Daily Journal and rate mood and any additional symptoms you may be experiencing from 1 to 10. Rate with number 1 being the worst and number 10 being no side effect or symptom remaining.

Take: 4 Ultimate Omega 3 softgels.

Time: First thing in the morning when you wake up, and around noon but before 4 pm.

After the rigors of Step 1, you will find Step 2 quick and easy. You are finished and ready to move to Step 3.

Step 3

- **Continue taking all supplements as established during Steps 1 and 2.**

Goal:

- Improved sleep.
- A vast reduction or elimination of anxiety.
- A lessening or elimination of other medication-induced side effects.

Supplements you will take:

- Essential Protein Formula.
- Body Calm.
- Body Calm Supreme.

Day One:

Action:

- Rate your daytime mood, anxiety, panic attacks, insomnia, fatigue and other side effects. Use the Daily Journal and rate anxiety, sleep and any additional symptoms you may be experiencing from 1 to 10. Rate with number 1 being the worst and number 10 being no side effect or symptom remaining.

Take: Essential Protein Formula: 1 teaspoon mixed in a liquid of your choice.

Body Calm Supreme capsule: 1 capsule.

Time: At bedtime.

Note: If you begin to feel tired during the daytime at any time during this Step, go back to the amount of Essential Protein Formula, Body Calm and Body Calm Supreme you were last taking before you felt tired. Remain at that level.

Day Two, Three, Four:

Action:

- Rate your daytime mood, anxiety, panic attacks, insomnia, fatigue and other side effects. Use the Daily Journal and rate anxiety, sleep and any additional symptoms you may be experiencing from 1 to 10. Rate with number 1 being the worst and number 10 being no side effect or symptom remaining.
- Rate the previous night's sleep first thing the next morning.
- Rate the daytime anxiety just before bedtime of that day.

Take: Essential Protein Formula: 1 teaspoon mixed in a liquid of your choice.

Body Calm Supreme capsule: 1 capsule

Time: First thing in the morning when you awake.

The rest of the day and up until bedtime, you will be alternating the Body Calm Supreme and the Body Calm every 4 hours.

Example: You awaken at 7 am. Start the day by taking 1 capsule of Body Calm Supreme and 1 teaspoon of Essential Protein Formula.

At 11 am, you would take 1 Body Calm capsule and 1 teaspoon of Essential Protein Formula.

At 3 pm, you would take 1 Body Calm Supreme capsule and 1 teaspoon of Essential Protein Formula.

At 7 pm, you would take 1 Body Calm capsule and 1 teaspoon of Essential Protein Formula.

At bedtime, or 11 pm, you would take 1 Body Calm Supreme capsule and 1 teaspoon of Essential Protein Formula.

Step 4

Day 1:

Begin taking 400 i.u. of vitamin E first thing in the morning. Take the vitamin E with the rest of the morning supplements.

Begin taking 1 capsule of Nature's Vitamin C any time around midday. (Do not take vitamin C if taking ADHD Medication.)

Other Options

If you are still feeling any depression, you can take up to 3 softgels of CLA daily. Take 1 in the morning, 1 near noon and the third softgel before 4 pm. CLA has been clinically proven to significantly stop the production of IL-6, a marker of depression.

If you have not added the Probiotic Supreme to your daily supplements, you might have Candida yeast overgrowth. Adding the Probiotic Supreme for 60 days may be just the assistance your body needs.

Your other option to further lower the IL-6 levels is with RenewPro. You can add up to 2 full scoops each day to your routine.

Keep taking all supplements exactly as you have established during the pre-taper.

You are completely finished with the pre-taper when:

- 22 days have passed after you started Step 1

    and

- You rate yourself at a 7 or higher for anxiety and sleep.

You do need to wait the 22 days from the date you started Step 1 before you begin the taper process.

Continue taking all of supplements exactly as you are now during the tapering portion of the program.

If you have tried to quit these medications in the past, you may be a little apprehensive about reducing the medication again. You can remain at this stage of the process for as long as you like. You do not have to rush.

When you are ready, follow the procedures detailed in the chapter, How to Taper off Cymbalta (Slow and Gradual Taper) or How to Taper off Cymbalta (Fast and Gradual Taper).

CHAPTER 11

HOW TO TAPER OFF BENZODIAZEPINES, ANTI-ANXIETY, ANTICONVULSANTS AND SLEEP MEDICATIONS
(SLOW AND GRADUAL TAPER)

Now that you have completed your pre-taper program, you are ready to start the reduction of your medication.

Though not knowing what you may have experienced personally, the vast majority of people who are ready for this step tell me that they have some trepidation starting the taper, due to terrible side effects when they have tried to quit before.

As incredible as it might seem, this step should be the *easy* part of The Road Back Program.

This tapering method is the Slow and Gradual Taper. It takes more time but the chance is extremely low of withdrawal side effects. You may wish to use this method the first 3 reductions, see you can successfully lower the medication this time and then move to the Fast and Gradual Taper.

The Taper
The *safest* method to reduce medication:

If you have tried to taper off these medications before and suffered withdrawal side effects, start the taper slowly. Successfully lower the medication by 2% every 14 days for three reductions, then move on to the next method for reducing the medication.

Some people have said that the 2% reduction every 14 days takes too long. My response, "How long have you been trying to get off the medication?" The answer was usually a few years without success. Tapering is where *slow, and steady* wins the race every time.

Again, if you had a problem in the past with tapering off medication, definitely use the 2% reduction schedule. Successfully reduce the medication at least 3 times. See for yourself that you can, and still feel well. Then you and your physician should decide if you should reduce the medication more quickly.

Make sure you work with the prescribing physician before changing the dosage of your medication.

Ask your physician to write a prescription to accommodate a 2% reduction. Use a compounding pharmacy to fill this prescription.

- It is important that the compounded drug be identical to the drug you are currently taking.

- Changing to a generic drug may not act the same, and withdrawal side effects can begin.

- Switching from one drug to another because it has a longer half-life will create withdrawal side effects caused by the drug abruptly stopped. Avoid this altogether.

- Unless the pharmacist can assure you that the medication is *exactly* the same, avoid this method of compounding.

- Only reduce the medication 2% every *fourteen days*. The 2% reduction is based on the original dosage of the medication. The 2% reduction is based on milligrams.

- Never skip any days of taking medication.

- Always take your medication at the same time each day.

- If you take your medication more than once each day, make sure the *total* reduction of the medication is no more than 2%.

- Take each supplement at least half an hour apart from the drug, but ideally, 1 hour apart. It is much better to take the supplements 1 hour after taking the drug, instead of before the drug.

- Continue with your supplements and "super foods" at the same times and amounts established during the pre-taper.

- Continue taking your "super foods" and supplements at least 45 days ***after*** you take the last dosage of your medication.

- Remember fill out you Daily Journal daily and keep taking all the supplements exactly as you did at the end of the pre-taper.

After 3 full reductions at the 2% reduction rate you can increase the taper to a 5% percent reduction of the medication every fourteen days.

Taper Procedure:

1. Keep taking all supplements exactly as you did at the end of the pre-taper throughout the taper process.

2. Keep your Daily Journal up to date each day.

3. Compound medication for a 2% reduction.

4. Reduce medication by 2% every 14 days, at least during the first 3 reductions.

5. Reduce the medication at the lowest possible amount, using the drug manufacturer's available tablet or capsule.

6. Reduce the medication every 14 days.

7. Make sure you have at least 7 consecutive days of feeling very well before reducing the medication again. If this requires you to reduce the medication every 21 days, do that.

8. Never skip any days of taking medication

Tapering can be this simple.

What to Do if Side Effects Begin

Withdrawal side effects can happen, but addressing them early and knowing what to do will usually make them short-lived and keep them mild as well.

"With little, to no side effects," is mentioned several times in this book, but a $250,000 automobile still comes with a spare tire, just in case.

If a Withdrawal Side Effect Turns On During the Taper:

Do not reduce the medication again until the symptom goes away. This usually takes a only few days or less, and then you can resume the taper.

Do not start making wholesale changes to your daily routine.

Proceed with the following steps, in the order presented. Once the withdrawal side effect is eliminated give yourself 7 days, and then continue with the taper.

1. Review your Daily Journal and look for changes you might have made to your routine. If you located a change, go back to exactly what you were doing before the change and all should soon be well. Give the withdrawal side effect 7 days to go away. If nothing is found, move to number 2.

2. Usually the withdrawal side effect will be a side effect you had before doing the pre-taper. Review the Daily Journal and locate the exact step of the pre-taper that eliminated the side effect.

   Increase that supplement slightly when taken during the daytime or at bedtime and this should handle the side effect quickly.

   Once the side effect is gone, wait 7 days before reducing the medication again.

   If the side effect is not eliminated, this needs to be looked at a few different ways before taking any new action.

   Do you still rate yourself at a 7 or higher on the 1-10 scale for anxiety, sleep and other feelings? If so, keep taking the slight increase of the supplement that handled the side effect previously for the next 7 days and then continue with the taper as long as you remain at a 7 or higher rating.

   - Each supplement used with The Road Back Program has a specific purpose.
     Using a supplement a little differently is sometimes needed to overcome withdrawal side effects.
     Begin taking the Body Calm Supreme every 4 hours during the day if not already doing that.
     Once the side effect is eliminated or reduced to the point of rating yourself at a 7 or higher again, wait 3 days and then reduce the Body Calm Supreme back to the amount you were taking.
     Make sure you keep taking all other supplements exactly as established during the pre-taper.
     If you have fallen below a 7 rating, proceed to number 3.

3. If you found that number 2 handled the side effect and the same side effect begins again with the next reduction, 1 day before you reduce

the medication increase that supplement slightly and stay on the increased amount for 4 days after you lowered the dosage.

This approach should help prevent the side effect from ever being present with future reductions.

4. If number 2 did not fully eliminate the side effect, give yourself a little additional time. Stay at the increased amount of the supplement that you increased doing number 2 and relief should come within 7 days.

5. Sometimes there is a bump in the road as you taper off a medication. Withdrawal side effects being with no rhyme or reason. You might have decreased the medication 6 times with ease, and after the seventh reduction a withdrawal side effect begins.

This usually goes away using the steps above, but sometimes persists.

There are two solutions: Reducing the medication once again or increasing the medication back up to the last dosage where you were doing well.

If you are going to increase the medication, give yourself at least 14 days before doing so. Give your body a chance to adjust. However, if the withdrawal side effect is unbearable, do not wait the 14 days, instead complete steps 1-4 above and then proceed with this option.

Increasing the medication back to the last dosage should be the first choice of the two options.

There are times when reducing the dosage handles the withdrawal side effect. For whatever reason, your body is reacting to that certain amount of medication, and nothing you do will get rid of the side effect except to go onto a different dosage, whether higher or lower.

If you went back up on the dosage of the medication to get relief, and withdrawal side effects started when you returned to the previous level, the answer is usually to reduce the medication again rather quickly and get to a new lower level. This new level would be just under the dosage where you were when withdrawal side effects started with the taper.

Consult your physician and keep him or her well informed as to how you are doing and *what you are doing*.

Once off the medication, make sure you keep taking the supplements for 45 days.

CHAPTER 12

HOW TO TAPER OFF BENZODIAZEPINES, ANTI-ANXIETY, ANTICONVULSANTS AND SLEEP MEDICATIONS
(FAST AND GRADUAL TAPER)

Congratulations. You have completed your pre-taper program, and are ready to start reducing your medication.

Though not knowing your personal experience, I do know that the vast majority of people ready for tapering experience trepidation because they have suffered terrible side effects when trying to quit before.

As incredible as this might seem, this step should be the *easy* part of The Road Back Program. Take a moment and look at how you felt before the pre-taper. Compare how you feel now that the pre-taper is complete. You can make it off the medication.

Up till now, the problem with getting off medication has been availability of the medication in dosages that would allow gradual reduction.

Several of the drug inserts suggest reducing the medication every 3 days. Such rapid and large drops in the medication result only in suffering.

To survive, we sometimes need to change the current environment or change ourselves.

The existing environment of available dosages has been a constant problem for successful tapering.

Either the drug manufacturers needed to make their medication in dosages that would accommodate a gradual reduction or a solution had to be found to allow for large reduction while averting withdrawal side effects.

Most medications can be compounded by a pharmacist. When compounding, a pharmacist makes a medication for you at an exact dosage.

Psychiatric medications cannot always be compounded to exact dosages without altering the structure, and with some of the medications being time release, large reductions are the only option.

Therefore, for survival, we need to change the environment and change ourselves as well. In this case, the change was improving The Road Back Program to accommodate medications that could not easily be gradually reduced by a small percentage.

The Road Back Program will always be improving. However, at this writing, the program has made a giant stride in handling the environment, or better stated, handling the problem of available dosages supplied by the drug manufacturer.

This breakthrough includes benzodiazepines, antidepressants, antipsychotics, sleep medications, ADHD medications and even medications prescribed in time release form.

What to Do

Two days before the first reduction you will need to increase specific supplements. You will use data from your pre-taper Daily Journal during this phase.

You will be increasing supplements to avoid withdrawal side effects from starting and to greatly reduce the chance of having any problem with tapering off the medication.

If a side effect begins during the taper, the odds are greatest that it will be a side effect you had before the pre-taper. Be ready for that and make sure those supplements you used during the pre-taper are increased.

Each individual is different but there are common withdrawal traits a high percentage of people will share. Those are addressed in this taper and the goal is to never let them start.

You need to be the judge with the use of some of the supplements during this part.

Example: If you had anxiety and insomnia before the pre-taper which is now handled, you will want to address that potential during the taper by increasing the supplements that handled it during the pre-taper.

If the Body Calm Supreme totally handled daytime anxiety by taking 1 capsule every 4 hours during the day, you should increase the Body Calm Supreme to 1 capsule every 2 hours before you reduce the medication.

How to Increase Supplements

Use your Daily Journal and look back at the pre-taper. Locate the supplement or supplements that made the largest positive change. Detailed below are how much you can increase each supplement. You will also find located within ( ) what each nutritional supplement is good for.

Body Calm (anxiety and insomnia) – If you feel the Body Calm was the supplement that handled the daytime anxiety or insomnia you can increase the Body Calm to once every 2 hours during the daytime and up to 3 capsules at bedtime for sleep.

Essential Protein Formula (anxiety and insomnia) – This nutritional supplement can be increased to 8 tablespoons per serving.

RenewPro (anxiety, energy and brightness) – You can increase the RenewPro to 1 full scoop 3 times a day.

Nature's Vitamin C (anxiety) – You can increase this vitamin C to 6 capsules a day. (Avoid vitamin C and other fruit if taking ADHD medication to avoid vitamin/drug interactions. This includes fruit as well as natural fruit drink.)

Probiotic Supreme (anxiety, fatigue and depression) – Do not increase beyond recommendation on the bottle.

Ultimate Omega 3 (fatigue, brain zaps, depression and head feelings) – You can increase up to 5 softgels in the morning and 5 softgels at noon. (Make sure you are taking 400 i.u. vitamin E daily if taking Omega 3.)

Vitamin E – Do not increase beyond the 400 i.u. a day.

CLA (anxiety and depression) – You can increase to 1 softgel in the morning, 1 at noon and 1 additional before 4 pm. (Make sure you are taking at least three Omega 3 and 400 i.u. vitamin E daily if you are going to use the CLA.)

Calsorption (brain zaps) – You can take 5 grams each day. There is no benefit taking more. Calsorption increases the absorption of calcium and can be helpful with side effects in the gut. CalesiumD is only recommended as a calcium supplement.

CalesiumD (brain zaps) – CalesiumD and Calsorption work together as a team. To achieve the highest potential calcium absorption Calsorption is needed. Take 800 mg of CalesiumD daily or the amount recommended by your physician.

All these nutritionals work quickly when they are what your body needs. Having them all on hand to draw from as needed is very beneficial.

Here is an example of how to increase the nutritional supplements 2 days before a medication reduction.

Scenario – At the end of the pre-taper you are taking the following supplements. Your major symptoms before the pre-taper were anxiety and insomnia.

- (1) Body Calm every 4 hour (alternating with the Supreme)
- (1) Beta 1, 3-D Glucan in morning

- (1) Body Calm Supreme every 4 hours (alternating with the Body Calm)
- (1) Teaspoon of Essential Protein Formula every 4 hours and at bedtime
- (2) Ultimate Omega 3 in am and 2 additional at noon
- (1) Vitamin E
- (1/2) Scoop of RenewPro 3 times a day

Example of how to increase supplements 2 days before taper:

- (1) Body Calm every 2 hours (alternating with the Supreme)
- (1) Body Calm Supreme every 2 hours (alternating with the Body Calm)
- (1) Teaspoon of Essential Protein Formula every 2 hours and at bedtime
- (3) Ultimate Omega 3 in am and 3 additional at noon
- (1) Vitamin E in morning
- (1) Scoop of RenewPro 3 times a day
- (1) CLA in the am, noon and 3 pm
- Probiotic Supreme in the morning (As directed on bottle label)
- (2) Beta 1, 3-D Glucan in the morning, 2 at noon and 2 before 4 pm
- (1) Scoop of Calsorption anytime in the day
- 800 mg of CalesiumD in morning

Five days after the medication is reduced, as long as there are no side effects or only very mild side effects, reduce the supplements down to the amount you were taking before the increase.

Wait 10 full days after you reduce the supplements, then increase again for 2 days and then reduce your medication. Again, five days after the medication is reduced, as long as there are no side effects or only very mild side effects, reduce the supplements back down to what you were taking before the increase.

Wait 10 full days after you reduced the supplements and then increase supplements again for 2 days and then reduce your medication.

Repeat this sequence until off the medication. Make sure to stay on the increased supplements for 5 full days after your final reduction of the medication.

Follow instructions in the chapter Once Off Medication to complete program.

Example:

You are taking 10 mg of a medication

1. Increase supplements 2 days before reduction of medication
2. First reduction is to 9.5 mg
3. 5 days after reduction of medication, lower supplements to previous amount if all is well
4. Wait 10 days
5. Increase supplements 2 days before next reduction of medication
6. Reduce medication to 9 mg
7. 5 days after reduction of medication, lower supplements to previous amount if all is well
8. Wait 10 days
9. Increase supplements 2 days before next reduction of medication
10. Reduce medication to 8 mg

11. 5 days after reduction of medication, lower supplements to previous amount if all is well

12. Wait 10 days

13. Increase supplements 2 days before next reduction of medication

14. Reduce medication to 6 mg

15. 5 days after reduction of medication, lower supplements to previous amount if all is well

16. Wait 10 days

17. Increase supplements 2 days before next reduction of medication

18. Reduce medication to 4 mg

19. 5 days after reduction of medication, lower supplements to previous amount if all is well

20. Wait 10 days

21. Increase supplements 2 days before next reduction of medication

22. Reduce medication to 2 mg

23. 5 days after reduction of medication, lower supplements to previous amount if all is well

24. You are now off the medication and should proceed to the chapter Once Off Medication

What to Do If Side Effects Begin During Taper

It is important to take action if side effects begin while tapering off the medication. While withdrawal side effects can happen, addressing them early and knowing what to do will usually keep them mild and short lived.

Use the following steps if side effects take place while tapering.

Do not reduce the medication again until the symptom goes away. However, if the new side effect or symptom is very mild you can continue with the tapering of the medication and remain on the schedule.

In the previous example, if a side effect were to start during # 7 you would not lower the medication again until at least 10 days and 7 full days of feeling very well. So if you did not begin to feel very well until day number 12 of the waiting period, you should wait a full 7 additional days before reducing the medication again.

If the side effect is not eliminated, look at a few options before taking any new action.

Do you still rate yourself at a 7 or higher on the 1-10 scale for anxiety, sleep and other symptoms? If so, continue with the taper schedule.

Each supplement used in this program has a specific purpose.

Sometimes using a supplement a little differently overcomes withdrawal side effects.

Anxiety – If you responded well to the Body Calm Supreme during the pre-taper, taking the Supreme every 2 hours during the daytime works well. Do not take the Body Calm during the daytime with this approach.

If the Body Calm was the nutritional supplement that helped the most with daytime anxiety you can increase the Body Calm to 2 or 3 capsules each time you take it during the daytime. You can take the Body Calm every 2 hours if needed.

The Beta 1, 3-D Glucan might be the answer. Increasing this supplement to 10 capsules each day is fine. Split the amount taken between morning, noon and later afternoon. If this is the right supplement for your needs, once the amount is increased you will feel the positive difference in 1 to 3 days.

Insomnia – Handle insomnia as quickly as possible. Increase the Body Calm, Body Calm Supreme or Essential Protein Formula as needed.

Again, the key is taking good notes during the pre-taper and making a list of which supplement handled which side effect.

Fatigue – Increasing the RenewPro will be the answer.

The Taper

Stage 1

Successfully reduce the medication by 5% every 14 days for two reductions, then move on to Stage 2. If not able to reduce by exactly 5%, reduce the medication as close to 5% as possible.

Once successful reducing the medication at least 2 times, you'll see that you can do this and still feel well. Then you and your physician should decide if you should reduce the medication at a larger percentage.

Make sure you work with your prescribing physician before changing medication dosages.

Ask your physician to write a prescription to accommodate a 5% reduction, or as close as possible. You may need a compounding pharmacy to fill this prescription.

Again, we are not in a speed race. Experience success and then move on to Stage 2.

- If you compound the medication it is important that the compounded drug is identical to the drug you are currently taking.

- Unless the pharmacist can assure you that the medication is *exactly* the same, avoid compounding.

- A generic drug may not act the same and withdrawal side effects can begin.

- Switching from one drug to another because it has a longer half-life will create withdrawal side effects from the drug abruptly stopped

- Only reduce the medication 5% every *fourteen days*. The 5% reduction is based on the original dosage of the medication. The 5% reduction is based on milligrams.

- Never skip any days of taking medication.

- Always take your medication at the same time each day.

- If you take your medication more than once each day, make sure the *total* reduction of the medication is no more than 5%.

- Take each supplement at least half an hour between taking the drug, but ideally, 1 hour apart. It is much better to take the supplements an hour after the drug, instead of before.

- Continue with your supplements and "super foods" at the same times and amounts established during the pre-taper. Only increase supplements if a side effect begins.

- Take each supplement at the same time each day.

- Fill out your Daily Journal each day and keep taking all the supplements exactly as you did at the end of the pre-taper unless an adjustment was needed to handle a withdrawal side effect.

- After you have reduced the medication twice during Stage 1 plus 14 days have passed since the second reduction and you are doing well, move on to Stage 2.

Stage 2

Taper Procedure:

- Keep taking all supplements exactly as you did at the end of Stage 1.
- Keep your Daily Journal up to date.
- Compound medication for a 10% reduction if possible or reduce the medication as near to 10% as possible, using the drug manufacturer's available tablet or capsule.
- Reduce medication by 10% every 14 days or as close to 10% as possible.
- Only reduce the medication every 14 days.
- Make sure you have at least 7 consecutive days of feeling very well before reducing the medication again.
- Never skip any days of taking medication

Tapering can be this simple.

Once you are off the medication, make sure you keep taking the supplements for 45 days.

CHAPTER 13

HOW TO TAPER OFF CYMBALTA
(SLOW AND GRADUAL TAPER)

Congratulations: Having completed your pre-taper program, you are now ready to start reducing the Cymbalta. Though not knowing what you might have experienced personally, I do know that the vast majority of people ready for this step feel trepidation because of terrible side effects experienced when they tried to quit Cymbalta in the past.

You might have experienced the "electrical zaps" in the head that are very common with stopping antidepressants, a return of depression, anxiety, fatigue, extreme aches and pain or even wound up in a mental hospital.

Incredible as this might seem, this step should be the *easy* part of The Road Back Program.

The Taper

The *safest* method to reduce Cymbalta tablets:

If you have tried to taper off Cymbalta before and suffered withdrawal side effects, start the taper slowly. Successfully reduce the Cymbalta by 10% every 14 days for three reductions – then move to the next method for reducing the medication.

People have told me that the 10% reduction every 14 days is far too slow. When I responded, "How long have you been trying to get off the medication?" the answer was usually a few years without success. This is where *slow and steady* wins the race every time.

Again, if you had a problem in the past with tapering off Cymbalta, use the 10% reduction schedule. Successfully reduce the Cymbalta at least 3 times, see for yourself that you can do this and still feel well, and then you and your physician should decide if you should reduce the Cymbalta at a larger reduction.

Make sure you work with the prescribing physician before changing the dosage of your medication.

- • Ask your physician to write a prescription to accommodate a 10% reduction. **You will need to use a compounding pharmacy to fill this prescription.**
- It is important that the compounded drug be identical to the drug you are currently taking.
- Changing to a generic drug may not act the same and withdrawal side effects can begin.
- Switching from one drug to another because it has a longer half-life will create withdrawal side effects from the drug abruptly stopped.
- Do not switch from a tablet or capsule form of the drug to a liquid.
- Do not switch from a time release to a tablet form or liquid form of the drug.
- Unless the pharmacist can assure you the medication is *exactly* the same, avoid the compounding method.
- Only reduce the medication 10% every *fourteen days*. The 10% reduction is based on the original dosage of the medication. The 10% reduction is based on milligrams.

HOW TO TAPER OFF CYMBALTA (SLOW AND GRADUAL TAPER)

- **Never skip any days taking Cymbalta.**
- Always take Cymbalta at the same time each day.
- If you take Cymbalta more than once each day, make sure the *total* reduction of the medication is no more than 10%.
- Take each supplement at least half an hour apart from the Cymbalta, but ideally, 1 hour apart. It is much better to take the supplements 1 hour after taking the Cymbalta, instead of before the drug.
- Continue with your supplements and "super foods" at the same times and amounts established during the pre-taper.
- Take each supplement at the same time each day.
- Continue taking your "super foods" and supplements at least 45 days *<u>after</u>* you take the last dosage of Cymbalta.
- Remember fill out your Daily Journal filled day and keep taking all of the supplements exactly as you were at the end of the pre-taper.

After reducing the Cymbalta by 10% 3 times you can increase the reduction for the remaining of the taper to a 20% reduction every fourteen days.

Taper Procedure:

1. Keep taking all supplements exactly as you did at the end of the pre-taper throughout the taper process.
2. Keep your Daily Journal up to date each day.
3. Compound the Cymbalta for a 10% reduction.
4. Reduce the Cymbalta by 10% every 14 days, at least during the first 3 reductions.
5. Only reduce the Cymbalta every 14 days.

6. Make sure you have at least 7 consecutive days of feeling very well before reducing the Cymbalta again. If this requires you to reduce the Cymbalta every 21 days, do that.
7. Never skip any days of taking Cymbalta.
8. After 3 successful reductions at 10% and fourteen days have passed begin reducing by 20% every 14 days.

Tapering Cymbalta can be this simple.

What to Do If Side Effects Begin

Withdrawal side effects can happen, but addressing them early and knowing what to do will usually keep them mild and short-lived.

"With little to no side effects" is mentioned several times in this book, but if you were to purchase a $250,000 automobile, it would still come with a spare tire just in case.

Use the following steps if side effects take place while tapering.

If a withdrawal side effect turns on during the taper.

Do not reduce the Cymbalta again until the symptom goes away. This takes usually only a few days, or less, and then you can resume the taper.

Do not start making wholesale changes to your daily routine.

Proceed with the following steps, in this order. Once the withdrawal side effect is eliminated, give yourself 7 days. Then continue with the taper.

1. Review your Daily Journal and look for changes you might have made to your routine. If you located a change, go back to exactly what you were doing before the change and all should shortly be well. Allow 7 days for the withdrawal side effect to go away. If nothing is found when reviewing your journal, move to number 2.

2. Usually, the withdrawal side effect will be a side effect you had before doing the pre-taper. Review the Daily Journal and locate the exact step of the pre-taper that eliminated the side effect.

The exception to this is with *antidepressants*. The "electrical zaps" tend to occur only when an antidepressant is reduced. Immediately increase the Ultimate Omega 3 at the first sign of a head symptom or the "electrical zap." Immediately increase the Ultimate Omega 3 to 5 softgels in the morning and 5 softgels at noon, if this side effect begins.

Usually, the side effect will subside the same day or the next day with the increase of the Ultimate Omega 3.

If you are not already taking the Calsorption and CalesiumD, you should begin doing so now to avoid any return of the "electrical zaps." Taking 5 grams of Calsorption daily along with 800 mg of CalesiumD daily is recommended throughout the rest of your taper and for 45 days after the last dosage of medication.

If the head side effect remains mild, but is still present, continue taking the 5 softgels of Ultimate Omega 3 until the symptom abates and then return to your previous amount of Ultimate Omega 3. Wait 7 full days and then continue with the taper.

If the head side effects are severe and you find it difficult to function in life due to the pain of the symptom, go back to the last dosage of the Cymbalta before this reduction and remain there for 14 days. Going back to the last dosage should get rid of the "electrical zaps" quickly.

The next time you reduce the Cymbalta and each reduction thereafter, increase the Ultimate Omega 3 to 5 softgels in the morning and 5 softgels at noon 2 days before you reduce the medication, and remain at this level for 5 days after reducing the Cymbalta. This approach should avert the occurrence of the "electrical zaps."

If the "electrical zaps" continue with this approach, you will need to lower the Cymbalta more slowly. Talk to your physician and get your pharmacist to find a way to fill the prescription to allow for a more gradual reduction. This will handle the taper for you.

Usually the withdrawal side effect will be one you had before doing the pre-taper. Review your Daily Journal and locate the exact step of the pre-taper that eliminated the side effect.

Increase that supplement slightly when you take it during the daytime or at bedtime, and this should handle the side effect quickly.

Once the side effect is gone, wait 7 days before reducing the medication again.

If the side effect is not eliminated, look it over a few ways before taking any new action.

Do you still rate yourself at a 7 or higher on the 1-10 scale for anxiety, sleep and other feelings? If so, keep taking the slight increase of the supplement that handled the side effect earlier for the next 7 days and then continue with the taper as long as you remain at a 7 or higher rating.

If you have fallen below a 7 rating, proceed to number 3.

- Each supplement used with The Road Back Program has a specific purpose.

  Using a supplement a little differently is sometimes needed to overcome withdrawal side effects.

  Begin taking the Body Calm Supreme every 4 hours during the day if you are not already doing that.

Once the side effect is eliminated or reduced to the point of rating yourself at a 7 or higher once again, wait 3 days and then reduce the Body Calm Supreme back to the amount you were taking.

Make sure you keep taking all other supplements exactly as established during the pre-taper.

3. If you found that number 2 handled the side effect, and the same side effect begins again with the next reduction, 1 day before you reduce the medication, increase that supplement slightly and stay on the increased amount for 4 days after you lowered the dosage.

This approach should help stop the side effect from ever being present with future reductions.

4. If number 2 did not fully eliminate the side effect, you will need to give yourself a little additional time. Stay at the increased amount of the supplement that you increased doing number 2, and relief should come within 7 days.

5. Sometimes you hit a bump in the road as you taper. There is no rhyme or reason to when withdrawal side effects. You might have decreased the medication 6 times with ease and at the seventh reduction, a withdrawal side effect begins.

This usually goes away using the steps above, but sometimes persists.

There are two solutions: reducing the medication once again or increasing the medication back up to the last dosage where you were doing well.

Give yourself at least 14 days before increasing the medication. Give your body a chance to adjust. If the withdrawal side effect is unbearable, do not wait the 14 days but complete all steps above and then proceed with this option.

Increasing the medication back to the last dosage should be the first choice from these two options.

There are times when reducing the dosage handles the withdrawal side effect. For whatever reason, your body is reacting to that amount of medication and nothing you do will get rid of the side effect except to be on a different dosage, whether higher or lower.

If, to get relief, you increased the dosage of the medication, and withdrawal side effects started again when you returned to this level, the usual answer is to reduce the medication again rather quickly and get to a new lower level.

Make sure you talk to your physician about this and keep him or her well informed as to how you are doing and *what* you are doing.

Once you are off the Cymbalta, make sure you keep taking the supplements for 45 days.

Read the chapter, "Once Off Cymbalta" and follow the ending program completely.

CHAPTER 14

HOW TO TAPER OFF CYMBALTA
(FAST AND GRADUAL TAPER)

Congratulations.

To survive, we sometimes need to change the current environment or change ourselves.

The existing environment of available dosages has been a constant problem for successful tapering.

Either the drug manufacturers needed to make their medication in dosages that would accommodate a gradual reduction or a solution had to be found that would allow for large reduction while averting withdrawal side effects.

With these medications, it is not always possible to compound them to exact dosages without altering the drug structure, and with some of the medications being prescribed as time release, large reductions are the only option. Therefore, for survival, we need to change the environment and change ourselves as well. In this case, it was improve The Road Back Program to accommodate medications that could not be gradually reduced by a small percentage.

The Road Back Program will always be a work in progress. However, at this writing, that work has made a giant stride in handling the environment or better stated, the problem of available dosages supplied by the drug manufacturer.

This breakthrough includes medications that simply do not allow for a gradual reduction of 10% or even 20%.

With your pre-taper complete and Daily Journal kept up to date, you should know which supplement caused each positive change and handled which side effect up to this step.

You will be using that information during the taper phase of the program to handle any withdrawal side effect, if one begins.

Work with your prescribing physician before changing the dosage of your medication.

What to Do

Two days before the first reduction you will increase specific supplements. During this phase, you will use data from your pre-taper Daily Journal.

You will be increasing supplements to prevent withdrawal side effects from starting and greatly reduce any chance of having a problem with tapering off the medication.

If a side effect begins during the taper, the odds are greatest that it will be one you had before the pre-taper. Be ready for such and increase those supplements you used during the pre-taper.

While each individual is different there are common withdrawal traits a high percentage of people will share. Those are addressed in this taper as well. The goal is ensure they never start.

You will need to judge the use of some of the supplements during this part.

Example: If you had anxiety and insomnia before the pre-taper and that is now handled, you will want to address that potential during the taper by increasing the supplements that handled it during the pre-taper.

If the Body Calm Supreme totally handled the daytime anxiety by taking 1 capsule every 4 hours during the daytime, you should increase the Body Calm Supreme to 1 capsule every 2 hours before you reduce the medication.

How to Increase Supplements

Using your Daily Journal and looking back at the pre-taper, locate the supplement or supplements that made the largest positive change. Here is how much you can increase each supplement. You will also find located within ( ) what each nutritional supplement addresses.

Body Calm (anxiety and insomnia) – If you feel the Body Calm was the supplement that handled the daytime anxiety or insomnia you can increase the Body Calm to once every 2 hours during the daytime and up to 3 capsules at bedtime for sleep.

Essential Protein Formula (anxiety and insomnia) – This nutritional supplement can be increased to 8 tablespoons per serving.

RenewPro (anxiety, energy and brightness) – You can increase the RenewPro to 1 full scoop 3 times a day.

Nature's Vitamin C (anxiety) – You can increase this vitamin C to 6 capsules a day. (Avoid vitamin C and other fruit if taking ADHD medication to avoid vitamin/drug interactions. This includes actual fruit as well as natural fruit drink.)

Probiotic Supreme (anxiety, fatigue and depression) – Do not increase beyond recommendation on the bottle.

Ultimate Omega 3 (fatigue, brain zaps, depression and head feelings) – You can increase up to 5 softgels in the morning and 5 softgels at noon. (Make sure you are taking 1 vitamin E daily if taking Omega 3.)

Vitamin E – Do not increase beyond the 400 i.u a day.

CLA (anxiety and depression) – You can increase to 1 softgel in the morning, 1 at noon and 1 more before 4 pm. (Make sure you are taking Omega 3 and vitamin E if you are going to use the CLA.)

Power Barley Formula (energy and brightness) – You can increase the Power Barley Formula to 1 scoop in the morning, 1 scoop at noon and 1 scoop before 4 pm. Make sure you are taking a vitamin E to get the full effect of this barley formula.

Calsorption (brain zaps) – You can take 5 grams each day. There is no benefit to taking more. Calsorption increases the absorption of calcium and can be helpful with side effects in the gut. It is only recommended you take CalesiumD as a calcium supplement.

CalesiumD (brain zaps) – CalesiumD and Calsorption work together as a team. To achieve the highest potential calcium absorption Calsorption is needed. Take 800 mg of CalesiumD daily or an amount recommended by your physician.

All of these nutritionals work quickly when they are what your body needs. Having all of them on hand to draw from as needed is very beneficial.

Here is an example of how to increase the nutritional supplements 2 days before a medication reduction.

Scenario – At the end of the pre-taper you are taking the following supplements and your major symptoms before the pre-taper were anxiety and insomnia.

- (1) Body Calm every 4 hour (alternating with the Supreme)
- (1) Beta 1, 3-D Glucan in morning
- (1) Body Calm Supreme every 4 hours (alternating with the Body Calm)
- (1) Teaspoon of Essential Protein Formula every 4 hours and at bedtime
- (3) Ultimate Omega 3 in am and 3 additional at noon
- (1) Vitamin E (400 i.u.)

- (1/2) Scoop of RenewPro 3 times a day

Example of how to increase supplements 2 days before taper:

- (1) Body Calm every 2 hours (alternating with the Supreme)
- (1) Body Calm Supreme every 2 hours (alternating with the Body Calm)
- (1) Teaspoon of Essential Protein Formula every 2 hours and at bedtime
- (5) Ultimate Omega 3 in am and 5 additional at noon
- (1) Vitamin E in morning (400 i.u.)
- (1) Scoop of RenewPro 3 times a day
- (1) CLA in the am, noon and 3 pm
- Probiotic Supreme in the morning (As directed on bottle label)
- (2) Beta 1, 3-D Glucan in the morning
- (1) Scoop of Calsorption anytime in the day
- 800 mg of CalesiumD in morning

If you are taking the Power Barley Formula in place of the RenewPro to handle fatigue, you would increase the Power Barley to twice the amount where you were when you finished the pre-taper.

Five days after the medication is reduced, as long as there are no side effects or only very mild side effects, reduce the supplements back to the amount you were taking before the increase.

Wait 10 full days after reducing the supplements and then increase supplements once again for 2 days and then reduce your medication. Again, five days after reducing the medication, as long as there are no side effects or only very mild side effects, reduce the supplements to what you were taking before the increase.

Wait 10 full days after reducing the supplements and then increase supplements once again for 2 days and then reduce your medication.

Repeat this sequence until off the medication. Make sure to stay on the increased supplements for 5 full days after your final reduction of the medication.

Follow instructions in the chapter Once Off Medication to complete program.

Example:

You are taking 60 mg of Cymbalta.

1. Increase supplements 2 days before reduction of medication
2. First reduction is to 40 mg
3. 5 days after reduction of medication, lower supplements to previous amount if all is well
4. Wait 10 days
5. Increase supplements 2 days before next reduction of medication
6. Reduce medication to 30 mg
7. 5 days after reduction of medication, lower supplements to previous amount if all is well
8. Wait 10 days
9. Increase supplements 2 days before next reduction of medication
10. Reduce medication to 20 mg
11. 5 days after reduction of medication, lower supplements to previous amount if all is well
12. You are now off the medication and should proceed to the chapter Once Off Medication

Increase the supplements 2 days before the reduction, keep taking the increased amount of supplements for 5 days after the reduction, wait 10 days and reduce the medication again.

What to Do If Side Effects Begin During Taper

While withdrawal side effects can happen, addressing them early and knowing what to do will usually keep them mild and short-lived.

Use the following steps if side effects take place while tapering.

Do not reduce the medication again until the symptom goes away. However, if the new side effect or symptom is very mild you can continue with the tapering of the medication and remain on the schedule.

In the previous example, if a side effect were to start during # 7 you would not lower the medication again for at least 10 days and 7 full days of feeling very well. So, if you did not begin to feel very well until day number 12 of the waiting period, you should wait 7 additional full days before reducing the medication again.

If the side effect is not eliminated, look at it a few ways before taking any new action.

Do you still rate yourself at a 7 or higher on the 1–10 scale for anxiety, sleep and other symptoms? If so, continue with the taper schedule.

Each supplement used in this program has a specific purpose.

Sometimes using a supplement a little differently is needed to overcome withdrawal side effects.

If you begin to get the "brain zaps" (electrical jolt that tends to run from the base of the neck to the base of the skull) address them by doing the following:

a. If you are not already taking 5 Ultimate Omega 3 in the morning and 5 at noon, begin doing so right away.

b. Make sure you are taking 1 vitamin E each morning

c. Begin taking 1 CLA softgel in the morning, 1 more at noon and 1 more before 4 pm.

d. Increase the RenewPro by half as much as you currently take

e. Start taking 2 Probiotic Supreme each day

f. Start taking 5 grams of Calsorption each day if you do not already take it

g. Start taking 800 mg of CalesiumD daily

It is important you handle the "brain zaps" quickly and fully.

Anxiety – If you responded well to the Body Calm Supreme during the pre-taper, taking the Supreme every 2 hours during the daytime works well. Do not take the Body Calm during the daytime with this approach.

If the Body Calm was the nutritional supplement that helped the most with daytime anxiety you can increase the Body Calm to 2 or 3 capsules each time you take it during the daytime. You can take the Body Calm every 2 hours if needed.

The Beta 1, 3-D Glucan might be the answer. Increasing this supplement to 10 capsules each day is fine. Split the amount taken between morning, noon and later afternoon. If this is the right supplement for your needs, once the amount is increased you will feel the positive difference in 1 to 3 days.

Insomnia – Handle the insomnia as quickly as possible. Increase the Body Calm, Body Calm Supreme or Essential Protein Formula as needed.

Again, the key is taking good notes during the pre-taper and making a list of which supplement handles which side effect.

Fatigue – Increasing the RenewPro or Power Barley Formula will be the answer.

CHAPTER 15

ONCE OFF CYMBALTA

Congratulations! If anyone ever deserved a celebration party for an accomplishment, it is you. You not only made it off Cymbalta, but also adhered to a schedule most other people have never had to confront. Only you can know what I mean.

As stated earlier in this book, you should continue taking all supplements for 45 days after the last dosage of the medication. It takes about 20 days for the enzymes used to metabolize the Cymbalta to return to a normal state, and depending on your own DNA, a certain amount of time for the Cymbalta to fully clear your body.

Continue writing in your Daily Journal during this ending of the program.

The supplements are not addictive and there is no withdrawal from these natural products. However, if you were lacking the nutrients found in a specific supplement and you discontinue using it, you may feel a letdown or a negative change. This would be the same feeling any person would have, even if they have never used Cymbalta.

Omega 3 is needed in our diet. The human body needs an adequate amount of vitamins, minerals, and amino acids from a food source to work at an optimum level.

All of the psychoactive medications affect our hormones, adrenals, and glucose tolerance. Read the chapter "The Road Back Science" for additional information.

Once off the Cymbalta for 45 days, it is advisable to get a complete physical exam with specific attention to hormones, adrenals, and glucose: an all-natural treatment, by a healthcare provider who fully understands that this intricate system is needed.

If You Suffered From Anxiety or Depression

I have searched for years to find an answer for what a person should do once off their medication. That search has now ended with finding the Depression Recovery Program. The underlying reason you went on the Cymbalta in the first place is probably still hanging with you to some degree. Being able to locate and eradicate the reason and any residual symptoms should be addressed.

Contact the Depression Recovery Program right away at 1-785-594-7070 or www.depressionrecoveryprogram.org for more information. I urge you to not wait on this but continue on to a full and complete return to life.

What to Do With Supplements

After you are off the medication for around 20 days, you may need to begin reducing some of the supplements.

Body Calm and Body Calm Supreme – If you begin to feel tired during the daytime, it may be time to lower the amount of *Body Calm or Body Calm Supreme* used during the daytime.

If you are going to lower either of these supplements during the daytime, lower the Body Calm first. Reduce slowly until the tiredness goes away. Keep your Daily Journal filled out each day. If the tiredness goes away by reducing or eliminating the daytime use of the Body Calm, keep taking the Body Calm Supreme exactly as you have been.

If tiredness persists, take the Body Calm Supreme every 6 hours, instead of every 4 hours during the daytime.

Another option is to begin taking or increasing the amount of Power Barley Formula during the daytime for tiredness.

If you were not able to take the Power Barley Formula during the pre-taper or were only able to take less than the highest amount indicated during the pre-taper, increase the Power Barley Formula instead of lowering the Body Calm or Body Calm Supreme.

Go back to the pre-taper chapter that applies to the medication you were taking and increase the Power Barley Formula as outlined in that chapter. Remember, this is powerful barley, only increase it until the positive change takes place. Continue with the Power Barley until you have finished at least one complete container.

Ultimate Omega 3 – If you are taking 4 of the Ultimate Omega 3 in the morning and at noon, you can reduce the Ultimate Omega 3 down to 3 softgels in the morning and 3 softgels around noon.

If any head symptoms reappear, increase the Ultimate Omega 3 back up.

Essential Protein Formula – Continue taking the Essential Protein Formula as you did during the pre-taper and taper process for 45 days.

Power Barley Formula – Keep taking the amount established during the pre-taper for the entire 45 days unless you begin to feel anxiety during the daytime. If you begin to feel anxiety during the daytime, decrease the Power Barley Formula by the same amounts it was increased during the pre-taper. Just reverse the process.

Vitamin E – Continue taking the 400 i.u. of vitamin E for the entire 45-days.

Beta 1, 3-D Glucan – If you had anxiety and or insomnia before tapering off the medication, the Beta 1, 3-D Glucan can be used as a maintenance supplement as needed.

After the 45 Days Have Passed

You can keep taking any and all of these supplements for life for general health if you wish. Many people do, who have never taken psychiatric medications.

In time you will probably find that you do not need to take as much of a supplement, or take a supplement as often, to maintain the good feeling you now have.

Once again, congratulations on completing The Road Back Program and may your journey in life from this point forward be ever-expanding.

CHAPTER 16

WHAT TO DO IF YOU HAVE ALREADY STARTED TO TAPER OFF CYMBALTA OR QUIT COLD TURKEY

The key to handling withdrawal side effects once you begin to reduce the Cymbalta is: **Put Control Back in the Process Again.**

Roughly 80% of the people who begin this program have already started to taper off Cymbalta and are experiencing withdrawal side effects. The recommendations or suggestions offered in this chapter come from years of experience assisting these individuals.

First, it is not YOU. **That may be difficult to grasp at first, but in time, you will come to understand it was not you; it was the withdrawal side effect.**

The First Decision, Do You

- Stay where you currently are on the Cymbalta and try to handle the withdrawal side effects and then continue with the taper once the side effects are gone?

- Go back up to the last dosage of the Cymbalta where you were doing better and hope the withdrawal side effects stop?

- Suffer through the withdrawal side effects and hope for the best?

- Begin taking an additional drug to try to mask the withdrawal side effects from the Cymbalta?

These are your four basic options. Choosing the correct course of action will determine your quality of life for the next several months or years. Work closely with your physician before making the decision.

Understanding how you probably feel and the urgency you most certainly have, time is of the essence. Talk to your doctor. If you cannot schedule an office visit within one day, call and speak with the physician, but alert your physician now.

What to Expect With Each Option

- **Stay where you currently are on the Cymbalta and try to handle the withdrawal side effects and then continue with the taper once they are gone?**

If you remain at the new dosage that started the withdrawal side effects and do nothing else, the withdrawal side effects will probably continue. Usually, allowing additional time to pass will not stop the withdrawal side effects. For the few who experience some relief by just allowing time, the relief was minimal and usually new side effects began as more time passed.

Depending on the severity of the withdrawal side effects, starting the pre-taper protocol for the Cymbalta should help. The time you have waited to begin the pre-taper nutritionals will usually determine how fast and how well you experience relief.

The normal response to starting the pre-taper nutritionals will be around seven days. You may feel some relief right away, but count on feeling the major positive changes around day number seven. Over the next few weeks, you should feel better each day.

Continue with the pre-taper protocol and once you have eliminated all or nearly all of the withdrawal side effects that were present, then, and only then, reduce the Cymbalta further.

- **Go back up to the last dosage of the Cymbalta you were doing better on and hope the withdrawal side effects stop?**

This option has been used by a few with success, but what usually happens is that the existing withdrawal side effects remain and additional side effects begin.

The correct course of action would be to use the pre-taper protocol and give yourself time to recover. You may not feel positive change for a few weeks, but relief should come if you just stay on the pre-taper.

The problem most people encounter with using this option is not feeling relief soon enough so they jump to something else, switch to a different medication, and add an additional medication to try and stop the existing withdrawal side effects.

The additional medication is regularly prescribed for anxiety and sleep. Usually, between one to two weeks after the new medication is started, it will no longer provide relief, but will increase the daytime anxiety and insomnia.

Use this option with caution.

If you have already taken this course of action, use the pre-taper for taking multiple medications. Ideally, you did not begin a third medication to try to handle the side effects from the two you are taking. If you have added a third, just follow the pre-taper, but expect to spend a little more time to get rid of all of the existing side effects.

- **Suffer through the withdrawal side effects and hope for the best?**

If the withdrawal side effects are very mild and you have been doing very well reducing the medication in the past, you might try doing nothing except remaining at the dosage where you currently are, wait until the withdrawal side effects stop then reduce the medication again further.

Some lucky people have "rolled a seven" and can simply reduce the Cymbalta without much problem and not suffer in the least.

- **Begin taking an additional drug to try to mask the withdrawal side effects from the Cymbalta?**

As earlier described, this choice has an extreme downside. You may experience some temporary relief, but will usually lose such in a short time and suffer new side effects from the additional medication. More medications will then be added to try to combat all of the new side effects. You wind up on a cocktail of medications, all being used to try to stop the negative reactions from the other medications.

Avoid this option unless it is a life-or-death situation.

If you have already taken this route, follow the pre-taper guideline, get rid of all or the majority of existing side effects and then taper the medications one by one.

Deciding which option to take will put control and predictability into the process for you and your physician. No matter which option you choose, control and predictability will take place once you knowingly choose an option.

The attempt here is to remove the guessing of "what is behind door number 1-4."

The odds are extremely high that you will make it through what you are currently experiencing. Knowing what to do next is 99% of the battle.

If You Quit the Medication Cold Turkey

If you found this book after stopping Cymbalta abruptly, you know what happens with that decision.

There is always a solution.

- Tell the prescribing physician what you have done. Please do this. Also tell the prescribing physician what you have read in these pages.

- If you have been off the Cymbalta for less than one week, it is suggested that you go back on the last dosage you were taking. Begin the pre-taper program for the Cymbalta and get stable once again. Then proceed with the program to taper off the Cymbalta.

- If you have been off the Cymbalta for more than 7 days, you are close to the point of no return regarding taking the Cymbalta again to get relief from the side effects.

If you go back on the Cymbalta the odds are high that the withdrawal side effects will not stop and a host of new side effects will begin. This information is not in the literature supplied by the drug manufacturer or medical journals. This data is based on communicating with thousands of individuals at this crossroad during the past years and what happened when they took a specific avenue.

Again, inform your physician about what you have done and share this information with the physician.

Start the pre-taper and give the pre-taper some time to work. It might take 14 days before you feel any relief, but the chances are very high that relief is obtainable.

Do not give up hope.

CHAPTER 17

HOW TO TAPER OFF MULTIPLE MEDICATIONS

"Thank you! Thank you! Thank you! I feel 100% better!!!! Oh My Gosh. I cannot believe how great I feel. I'm actually getting ME back. I can see my personality, my spunk, my spark increase gradually each and every day, more and more. I cannot thank you enough. This has changed my life dramatically!

Please let me know how I can help to talk with others, to educate them, encourage them on getting their lives back and not depending on these drugs.

I know I still have a long way before I am completely healed. I look at it like this, though. If I feel this great now and I've only been off these 2 drugs (Klonopin and Cymbalta) for about 2 1/2 weeks, I cannot wait to see how I'll be feeling a month from now. I thought I'd never get over that dizzy, lightheaded, floating feeling in my head, with the lack of concentration and the agonizing pain in my joints and muscles.

Each day has gotten easier and easier. I had some very hard ones in there, though, but I am so happy I have done this.

The other day, I was teaching a Boot camp class and I had a coat on that I hadn't worn since last fall, I put my hand in my pocket and there was a Klonopin in there. I looked at it and it really made me think. A month ago, if I was in that stressful class situation I would have taken a small bite out of that little pill...instead I threw it away!!!!!

I really am serious about wanting to spread the word about these drugs. I think everything happens for a reason and there's a season for everything. This was the right time for me to stop taking them. I just want others who depend on these medications to be aware and know more of what the doctors are not telling us. Again thank you for helping me get my passion back"

"Today has been the 5th day on the supplements. 10 days with no Klonopin! 12 days with no Cymbalta! I am feeling a lot of relief from the dizziness/brain zaps and concentration or lack of. Thank God, because that is the worst withdrawal symptom!! I'm sleeping better, very deep and feel very rested. My appetite has decreased YEAH!!! Thank you!!!"

"I read through your site for about one month before trying the products myself. I must say, all of the "Oh, God's" in your testimonials made me wonder if this could really be true. I was told not to really expect a change for 3 to 7 days. After day 1 I had to call TRB Health and tell them what they had here. The "Oh, God" statements I have read now make sense. I was taking an antidepressant and a benzodiazepine and reached the state of no energy, a grinding anxiety during the day, could not sleep at night and more. The Power Barley Formula and the cherry blew me away. You guys have a spokesperson when you want one. Thank you."

What to Do If You Are Taking Multiple Drugs

If you are taking a benzodiazepine, anti-anxiety or sleep medication along with Cymbalta, deciding which medication to first taper off is important. There are times when a benzodiazepine or sleep medication will have a drug/drug interaction with Cymbalta, anti-psychotics and ADHD medications.

Most of the time an antidepressant, anti-psychotic or ADHD medication **_will_** have a drug-drug interaction with other antidepressant, anti-psychotic or ADHD medication ...but not always. Which drug you wean yourself from first will be largely responsible for your success.

The most common reason these medications have a drug/drug interaction is that they share the same metabolizing route. Two medications trying to go through the same pathway will create a "cumulative" effect of the medications and usually one or both medications will take longer to clear the body.

Imagine 4 linemen from your favorite football team trying to push through the front door of your home, shoulder to shoulder. None of the linemen will back off and let the other pass through first. This is what is happening inside the body.

Occasionally, one medication will _greatly_ increase the effect of another medication.

If you are taking a benzodiazepine with Cymbalta the benzodiazepine will be increased slightly due to the Cymbalta. If you begin to lower the Cymbalta you will also have a slight lowering of the benzodiazepine. Valium is the one exception to this as Valium metabolizes using a different route and is not affected by the Cymbalta.

If you are taking an antipsychotic or ADHD medication with Cymbalta, all of the medications use the same metabolizing route to some degree and they will also be reduced if you begin to lower the Cymbalta.

You should use the slow and gradual taper method if you are taking other psychoactive medication with Cymbalta.

If taking a benzodiazepine along with Cymbalta, use the pre-taper outlined for Cymbalta.

When reducing any of the medications, use the instructions found for that class of medication. Wait 14 days before reducing the next medication.

Continue taking all supplements as established during the pre-taper.

CHAPTER 18

WHAT CAN BE DONE IF YOU HAVE NEVER TAKEN PSYCHIATRIC MEDICATION

If you are suffering from anxiety, stress that does not seem to end, fatigue or a host of symptoms, you absolutely have an alternative to psychiatric medication.

First: Get a complete physical and have the physician rule out all disease or illness.

There can be life events that were the direct cause of depression, anxiety, stress, fatigue and more. Usually, these feelings go away on their own in a matter of days or weeks without you doing anything other than letting some time pass.

These medications are strong, some are truly addicting, and all of the drugs are life altering. The question is how your life will be altered.

When depression, anxiety, stress, and/or fatigue begin, other factors also play a role in general health. Levels of hormones, adrenals, glucose, cortisol and other functions can become drained, imbalanced or overly stimulated. Psychoactive medications, in part, are designed to regulate all of these functions to some degree, but they ultimately affect these functions by altering other chemicals in the brain and body.

Second: If you are diagnosed with a disease or illness, make sure the diagnosis is from an objective test – not a subjective analysis. As of this writing, all mental disorders are diagnosed with subjective tests.

Later in this chapter you will find possible solutions for symptoms you may be experiencing. One example is using the Body Calm, Body CalmSupreme and Essential Protein Formula for anxiety symptoms. These supplements do not cure disease or illness. With that in mind, **if** you feel the anxiety vanish once you begin using these supplements, you must not have had an Anxiety Disorder.

If you were diagnosed with chronic fatigue syndrome, take the Power Barley Formula and vitamin E, and no longer feel the fatigue, you were misdiagnosed. Misdiagnoses can and do happen.

If a diagnosis of ADHD is presented, then you take Ultimate Omega 3, vitamin E, and possibly Body Calm and your symptoms subside, you did not have ADHD. Again, these supplements do not cure or prevent disease or illness. If you feel the major positive changes after using these supplements, your body was just lacking those nutrients.

Good-meaning, well-intentioned physicians often feel like they must prescribe psychoactive medication or face the threat of malpractice. One senior partner in a law firm refused to even read this book. Why? His answer was, "If there is a way to taper off psychiatric drugs, with little to no side effects, we would no longer have a case."

If you receive a clean bill of health from your physician, there are suggestions and probable solutions.

Anxiety Stress, Fatigue, and Depression – Anxiety, stress, fatigue and depression quickly wear the body down. In no time the body begins to feel drained and rundown. One can easily lose track of where the anxiety, stress, fatigue or depression started, and when the body seemed to lump together with your overall feeling.

The goal of The Road Back is to assist you in keeping you separated from the anxiety, stress, fatigue and depression from the body.

As an example, take a finger on your hand.

You can unintentionally hit your finger with a hammer. Your hurt finger will have an effect on you until it heals. You can also decide to hit your finger with a hammer and have an effect on your body.

In either case, if the finger were hit hard enough, you and the injured body part would begin to lump together and you would begin to feel like you were only the body. Or your attention would become so fixed on the body that it would be difficult to distinguish the two. Your entire attention becoming fixated on the hurt finger.

Ask an artist to hit his/her finger with a hammer very hard and to then paint a beautiful picture or create anything not associated with pain. It will not happen. The live, creating part of us, the part that feels emotion – both wanted or unwanted emotion – begins to collapse with the body.

There is not a drug made that can prevent a person from hitting his or her finger with a hammer.

If you have just lost a loved one, or on a lesser scale, just lost your job, there are no supplements or medications that will replace the loss.

The most a psychoactive medication will do is deaden the feelings experienced because of the loss. The most a good supplement will do is assist the body to not succumb to the continued drain put on it because of the feeling of loss.

The Road Back has zero chance of coming into your life and handling the life reason for anxiety, stress, depression or even fatigue. However, we can assist your body to not succumb to the physical stressors being put on it daily from emotional trauma.

Hundreds of clinical trials have shown that people with anxiety; stress, fatigue and depression have low levels of amino acids, vitamins, minerals, antioxidant levels and more. These clinical trials point to the fact that a person will suffer a depletion of these vital nutrients if they are put under enough stress or duress for a period of time.

Our goal here is to point out a few things you can do to help your body maintain general health and well-being while you address the real reason for the problem you are experiencing.

When using the terms anxiety, stress, depression and fatigue, we do not imply a disease or illness associated with these conditions.

If you are trying to choose between two different jobs or changing jobs and feel anxiety and stress, that anxiety or stress is not a disease. After choosing one or the other, the anxiety or stress would vanish. If you just experienced a loss in life, that loss is not a disease. That is part of what eventually happens to each living person. Natural emotions are not diseases or illnesses. You should be considered very sane and normal.

If an emotion continues beyond some arbitrary "they should be over it by now" time period, psychoactive medication comes into play. Neither these drugs nor supplements will help you "realize" or have a "earth shattering realization" about why you have felt that way for such a long time or remove the loss you feel. **They will not.**

Psychoactive medication may block the emotion, but the emotion will need to be dealt with at some time in the future, unless you just wish to feel "flat-lined" forever. Most people tell us, in hindsight, they would have been better off dealing with the emotion when it happened, instead of putting it of for months or years and then dealing with the emotion on top of the drug withdrawal.

This is why The Road Back suggests using a few supplements. Again, the supplements are not going to solve the problem or underlying condition. They will only help maintain the body's general health and well-being and give you the chance to address the original problem.

We break down symptoms into two areas; anxiety/stress/insomnia, or fatigue. You may feel that you have depression, but even the depression will fit in to one of these two categories.

For Anxiety/Stress/Insomnia: Go to the chapter General Pre-Tapering and Tapering Instructions and read the entire chapter. Then go to the chapter

Pre-Taper for Benzodiazepines, Anti-anxiety, Anticonvulsant and Sleep Medication and follow the pre-taper instructions.

Use the Daily Journal and complete the entire pre-taper. This should handle all anxiety, stress and /or insomnia, if present. You can use these supplements as long as you wish; they are not addictive or habit forming.

For Fatigue: Read the entire chapter General Pre-Tapering and Tapering Instructions. Then go to the chapter Pre-Taper for Cymbalta and follow the pre-taper instructions in the section, *If You Have Fatigue*.

CHAPTER 19

THE SCIENCE BEHIND THE ROAD BACK

INTRODUCTION

The Road Back Program and the Development of the Program:

1. There are basic common denominators of psychotropic drug side effects.

2. How our individual DNA affects drug metabolism.

3. The effect of psychotropic medication within the Hypothalamus-Pituitary-Adrenal Axis and immune system.

4. Utilizing DNA clinical trials, test subject trials and psychotropic drug clinical trials to formulate specific nutritional products to eliminate, reduce or avert withdrawal side effects, while not creating drug/supplement interactions.

This research and development complexity has been transformed into an easy to understand, systematic program, which allows an individual to taper off their medication while alleviating a vast percentage of the debilitating side effects of withdrawal.

The sequence of this program and the application of each step is the key to success. Your patient will not even begin to reduce Cymbalta until all, or nearly all, existing Cymbalta-induced side effects are eliminated. This gives the physician as well as the patient, prediction, as well as a structured step-by-step standard approach for tapering off psychoactive medication.

Statements of fact: All psychoactive medications metabolize through specific pathways. *All* psychoactive medications alter the Hypothalamus Pituitary-Adrenal Axis to some degree. To some extent, you can predict the duration before drug-adverse reactions begin with most psychoactive drugs; if the patient's P450 (CYP) enzymes have been screened.

A poor metabolizer as well as an extensive metabolizer will eventually reach the same saturation point; the poor metabolizer much faster, of course.

If one were to look at the basic structure of the human body, the chemical structure of psychiatric drugs, and include how psychiatric drugs are metabolized, how foods, vitamins, minerals, DNA, amino acids, hormones, glands, proteins, fatty acids and enzymes work, in relation to psychiatric drugs, you have The Road Back Science.

DNA and Prediction of Drug Adverse Reactions

The following charts detail the P450 enzymes used to metabolize the most common antidepressants, anti-psychotics, benzodiazepines and ADHD stimulant medications. An X in the row denotes that the medication utilizes that specific pathway. Below each chart, you will find other routes of metabolism if applicable.

These medications *inhibit* metabolism via listed CYP pathways.

Drug	P450 Enzyme Pathway				
Antidepressants	1A2	2C19	2C9	2D6	3A
Anafranil	X	X		X	X
Celexa		X		X	
Cymbalta	X			X	
* Elavil	X	X		X	
Effexor				X	X
Lexapro		X		X	
* Luvox	X	X	X	X	X
Pamelor				X	X
* Paxil	X	X	X	X	
* Prozac	X	X	X	X	X
Remeron	X			X	X
Sarafem	X	X	X	X	X
Strattera		X		X	
* Tofranil	X	X		X	X
Trazodone				X	X
* Wellbutrin	X		X	X	X
* Zoloft	X	X	X	X	X

These marked medications (*) will also use other routes for metabolism:

Elavil – UGT1A4, UGT1A3, P-gp

Luvox – 2B6, P-gp, intestinal 3A

Paxil – 2B6, P-gp

Prozac – 2B6, P-gp

Tofranil – UGT1A4, UGT1A3, P-gp

Wellbutrin – 2E1, 2A6, 2B6

Zoloft – UGT2B7, UGT1A4, P-gp, 2B6

Drug	P450 Enzyme Pathway				
Anti-psychotics	1A2	2C19	2C9	2D6	3A
Abilify				X	X
* Clozaril	X	X	X	X	X
* Geodon	X				X
* Haldol	X			X	
* Risperdal				X	X
* Seroquel					X
* Zyprexa	X			X	
Other					
Cogentin				X	
* Lithium					

These marked medications (*) will also use other routes for metabolism:

Clozaril – FMO, UGT1A4, UGT1A3

Geodon – Aldehyde oxidase substrate

Haldol – Glucuronidation, P-gp

Risperdal – P-gp, renal extraction

Seroquel – Glucuronidation, P-gp, intestinal 3A, epoxide by quetiapine

Zyprexa – Glucuronidation, FMO, UGT1A4.

Drug	P450 Enzyme Pathway				
Benzodiazepine Anti-anxiety Sleep Medication	1A2	2C19	2C9	2D6	3A
Ambien	X		X		X
Ativan	UGT2B7				
* BuSpar				X	X
* Depakote	X	X	X		X
Klonopin					X
Librium					X
* Valium		X			X
* Xanax		X			X

These marked medications (*) will also use other routes for metabolism:

BuSpar – Intestinal 3A
Depakote – UGT2B7, UGT1A6, UGT1A9, UGT2B15, UGT1A4, UGT1A3
Valium – 2B6, UGT2B7, intestinal 3A
Xanax – Hepatic 3A.

Drug	P450 Enzyme Pathway				
Stimulants	1A2	2C19	2C9	2D6	3A
Adderall				X	
* Concerta				X	
Dextrostat				X	
* Ritalin				X	

These marked medications (*) will also use other routes for metabolism:

Concerta – Glucuronidation.
Ritalin – Glucuronidation.

How to Use Charts to Decide Sequence of Medication Reduction

If you have two or more medications sharing the same CYP pathway to metabolize, reduce the medication that uses the fewest shared pathways first.

Example: If you are taking Cymbalta and Abilify, you would need to reduce the Abilify first.

If taking two antidepressants concurrently, or taking an antidepressant and an antipsychotic, selecting which one to reduce first would also follow the format outlined earlier in this section. The drug using fewer *common* CYP pathways should be reduced first.

If taking two antidepressants or one antidepressant and one antipsychotic, and the CYP pathways match, evaluate the current side effects, when each side effect started, when each medication was introduced, and determine from those side effects which taper schedule to follow.

From time to time, a person will also be taking a drug as an inducer of the CYP pathways.

Determine if this "inducer" was prescribed to help offset the inhibitor drug's effect or is the *inducer* drug prescribed for other health reasons not related.

You will generally find that those who are also taking the *inducer* medication will be suffering from a wide variety of adverse side effects. When reducing any medication attached to the same pathway as an inducer medication, reduce the normal taper speed by one-half for at least the first 2 months.

You may need to alternate reduction of the inducer drug and the inhibitor drug every other reduction in order to maintain a balance.

Other medications must be closely evaluated. Lipitor, as an example, is an inhibitor of the CYP 2C19, 2D6, and 3A, along with inhibiting the UGT1A3, UGT1A1, P-gp, and intestinal 3A.

Use drug product insert to determine metabolism route or the Physicians' Desk Reference.

Example 1: If taking multiple medications and each medication uses the same metabolic route, each of the medications is competing for clearance. If one medication is reduced, the other medications will also be reduced or clear the body faster.

Decide which medication to taper off first based on:

- CYP charts
- full evaluation of side effects
- when side effects started with which medication.

If patient has used Lexapro for two years and used Risperdal for 2 months and side effects increased dramatically once Risperdal was introduced, taper the Risperdal first.

Example 2: If multiple medications are being taken and all medications can metabolize through several routes, the impact will be lessened, and selecting which medication to taper first would not be pathway dependant.

- Avoid all *supplements* that compete with the same pathways, and eliminate as much as possible all foods that compete with the medication by inducing or inhibiting the metabolism routes of the medications.

Supplements, Herbs and Foods

Supplements, herbs or certain foods can have a direct impact on the success of the taper.

Datum: If a person smokes or drinks coffee before starting the pre-taper, do not suggest they quit. Cigarette smoke *induces* the CYP1A2, 2E1, 3A and UGT2B7. Nicotine inhibits UGT1A1, UGT1A4, UGT2A6, and UGT1A9. If taking Depakote and starting or stopping smoking, the impact on the medication will be dramatic

Coffee or caffeine inhibits the CYP1A2, 2E1 and the 3A. A high percentage of these medications metabolize through these pathways and caffeine usage will dramatically increase the medication, or if the person were to quit drinking caffeine, they would begin to go into withdrawal to some degree because the pathways will begin to metabolize the medication faster.

If you drink coffee and smoke along with Cymbalta, the Cymbalta metabolism will be altered. If you quit smoking or drinking coffee you will probably experience a Cymbalta adverse reaction. Quitting coffee and smoking may be a good thing to do for your health, but wait until completely off the Cymbalta for 45 days before quitting these other substances.

Broccoli, Brussels sprouts and cauliflower are excellent vegetables to consume, however, this type of vegetable will alter the metabolism rate of Cymbalta. Eat these vegetables in moderation only.

The times a person takes medication and when they drink two cups of coffee can have an impact as well. If the person drinks two cups of coffee every morning about one hour after their medication, and they change the time of the morning they drink the coffee, expect a slight to above average side effect from the medication.

Green tea, with its current popularity is the most problematic at this time. I am not saying green tea is not beneficial. I am saying there is a time and place for supplements, herbs and some specific foods once a person is off all medication for 45 days.

The person's current daily routine should not be changed. If they were on a poor diet before starting this program, do not change their diet drastically. If they did not exercise before starting this program, do not advise them to do more than a casual walk.

Once off all medication for 45 days, a healthy diet can be implemented, an exercise program that matches their current physical condition can be started, the patient can stop smoking, etc.

DNA Drug Reaction Testing and Taper Prediction

For the past several years, DNA drug reaction testing has been available to determine the patient's ability to metabolize medication through the CYP450 enzymes.

I have conducted over 200 drug reaction tests with the objective of determining how well drug-adverse reactions could be predicted, and if there were clinical use of this DNA data for tapering.

Prediction of a drug-adverse reaction: The individuals who were slow or poor metabolizers or hyper metabolizers experienced drug-adverse reactions faster than normal or intermediate metabolizers.

However, the normal or intermediate metabolizers still experienced adverse drug reactions, but after longer usage of the medication. *The metabolism type of the individual was not indicative of the severity of adverse reactions or duration.* Once the drug had saturated the CYP enzyme used for metabolism, all the individuals experienced the same side effect profile regardless of their metabolism speed noted from the DNA drug reaction test.

The test results from the DNA drug-reaction test did not lead to a worthwhile taper guide. It was postulated; if you were to induce the enzymes or inhibit an enzyme to match a specific test result and medication, you would be better able to adjust the metabolism and avoid withdrawal, or predict the withdrawal sequence. Again, this did not assist in tapering or eliminating withdrawal side effects in the slightest. This seems to parallel the results using an *inducer* drug to counteract the inhibition of the main drug.

If a DNA drug-reaction test has any use to a physician, it would be for predicting the dosage of the medication Coumadin. The initial prescription could be limited to a narrow band, and the correct therapeutic dosage would be found in a few weeks, instead of several months.

Nutritional DNA Test

Nutritional DNA testing provided this program substantial information to work with. I tested the ability of over 100 subjects to metabolize B vitamins, folate, calcium, Omega 3, phase II liver detox genes, and an assortment of other genetic differences that ultimately determine overall health and physical well being.

The Road Back Program and all suggested nutritionals used for medication tapering address the most common genetic variations of the population at large. Though DNA science is not precise at this date, enough evidence is available to formulate part of a program to address the highest percentage of the population.

Hypothalamus-Pituitary-Adrenal Axis (HPA)

Psychoactive medications play havoc with the HPA. While benzodiazepines usually help with anxiety for a certain time period, the feedback loop sending incorrect data will eventually cause cortisol levels to increase, and the result will be increased anxiety in the morning and mid-afternoon. Insomnia will usually follow the cortisol level increase. Other psychoactive medications have their own unique side effect profile and ultimate effect upon the HPA.

First year medical school textbooks describe hypothalamus as: "Hypothalamus is homeostasis or maintaining the body's status quo." As an example, blood pressure, body temperature, fluid, the electrolyte balance and body weight are held in a precise value labeled the "set-point." The body's set-point may change over time, but from day to day, the set-point will remain nearly fixed. With the HPA receiving continual input about the state of the body and the ability of the HPA to initiate changes, as anything might sporadically fall out of balance, it is vital for the HPA to have at hand all necessary nutrients to assist with the compensation.

When the HPA is out of balance, you will have a problem with insulin, stress, anxiety, weight gain, thyroid problems, fatigue, unbalanced sexual hormones and countless other body difficulties.

The hormone, ACTH, will eventually become out of balance, as will the other hormones and adrenals.

Psychoactive medication directly alters specific areas within the HPA. Examine any patient using psychoactive medication for more than three months and you will probably find a problem with hormones, thyroid, adrenals, cortisol and immune system or other areas within the HPA.

However, it will be equally important to move beyond the normal view of the HPA. Psychoactive medication side effects are quite varied and diverse. This is not to rehash data from medical school, but to tie in the knowledge gained in the educational process with psychoactive medication.

Some fibers from the optic nerve go directly to a small nucleus within the hypothalamus (suprachiasmatic nucleus). This nucleus regulates circadian rhythms, and couples the rhythms to the light/dark cycles.

The nucleus of the solitary tract will collect sensory data from the vagus and relay the data to the hypothalamus. This data will include blood pressure and gut enlargement.

The reticular formation receives a vast supply of inputs from the spinal cord and relays that data to the hypothalamus. Part of that data will be skin temperature.

Nuclei, circumventricular organs, are unique in their own right as they lack a blood-brain barrier. They monitor substances in the blood and have the ability to monitor substances normally shielded by the neural tissue. Here you will find regulation of fluid and electrolyte balance, by controlling thirst, sodium excretion, blood volume regulation and vasopressin secretion. Include in this the area postrema, and you have the detection of blood toxins and the vomit-inducing center. The OVLT and area postrema project to the hypothalamus.

The limbic and olfactory systems project to the hypothalamus. Psychoactive medication side effects, such as eating problems and reproduction difficulty, will probably be traced to this area.

Ionic balance and temperature will be subject to the hypothalamus via the receptors, thermoreceptor and osmorecepter.

When the hypothalamus is aware of a problem, it will assert repair mechanisms. Neural signals to the autonomic system will attempt to regulate heart rate, vasoconstriction, digestion, sweating etc, and the endocrine signals to and or through the pituitary.

The pituitary side effects will include one or all six hormones, to include ACTH and the thyroid-stimulating hormone (TSH).

The repair output attempt, and the psychoactive medication side effect profile, seem to run near a 50 percent occurrence. Furthermore, you can directly trace psychoactive medication side effects to the autonomic nervous system in both the sympathetic and parasympathetic systems.

The hypothalamus can alter blood pressure; control every endocrine gland in the body, body temperature, adrenal levels via ACTH, and metabolism.

The repetition of HPA information in this chapter has been intentional. Do not be surprised to find a male patient with extremely high estrogen levels, a female with high testosterone or any other problem that can be associated within the HPA.

Taper the medication first, wait 45 days after the last dosage of the medication, reevaluate the patient, and then gradually bring all parts of the HPA back into balance. The nutritionals used with The Road Back Program were developed to help the body overcome this imbalance *gradually*. Gradually is italicized because this is where most problems occur with psychoactive drug-taper programs. Either they do not address the HPA or the program is really a detoxification or heavy metal chelating program.

The Road Back Program utilizes specific nutritionals to address the drug side effects and to begin the process of balancing the HPA. Specifics on each nutritional, what each nutritional is addressing within the HPA or the body in relation to psychoactive medications, can be found in The Road Back Program patent when published by the U.S. Patent Office.

Immune System

The immune system and the HPA are in constant communication and actions within one system will induce response in the other. The supplements used in this program are designed to also influence the immune response.

Interleukin-2 (IL-2) can be increased and anxiety, psychotic behavior, insomnia and other assorted manifestations associated with these symptoms may very well vanish. Beta 1, 3-D Glucan is clinically proven to increase IL-2 levels in humans.

When using the IL-2 reference range of 223-710 as a guideline, keep in mind any result with IL-2 lower than 466 needs to be increased if still showing signs of anxiety, psychosis or insomnia. It is advantageous to test the IL-6 along with the IL-2 for a complete understanding of the person's current immune response and inflammation factors.

IL-6 reference range will be from 0.0 – 14.0. If the IL-6 is greater than 3, it is advantageous to gradually lower the inflammation. Those with a low

IL-2 and high IL-6 will fall in the category of highly anxious and fatigued or depression symptoms.

Titrating Medication

The Road Back has tried titrating medication gradually without the use of nutritionals and limited success. 50% of the people could taper off their medication but they suffered extreme withdrawal side effects.

Using a gradual titration combined with a basic detoxification approach had lower than 50% success.

The normal supplements used to remove heavy metal or for a liver detox produced undesirable results.

A gradual titration with the use of the suggested nutritionals gives the standard results.

The Key to a Successful Taper With The Road Back Program

Following the pre-taper exactly as described is critical. The pre-taper is the make or break point for *every* successful taper. Setting the body up nutritionally and getting rid of all, or the vast majority of, existing side effects needs to be accomplished so the person knows they can make it off the medication and allow them to reduce the medication without causing additional trauma.

Most problems occur when:

- The pre-taper is done too quickly.
- Patient does not stop increasing a nutritional once a positive change occurs.
- Patient changes the time of day they take medication.
- Patient changes the time of day they take nutritionals.

- Medication is reduced too quickly.
- A new medication is prescribed in addition to existing medication.
- Patient is switched to a new medication.
- Doctor has patient use additional supplements or vitamins not in this program.
- Patient begins taking other supplements.
- Patient makes a major change to their daily routine.
- Patient skips day of taking medication.

Additional Items

When you have a patient taking a vast array of vitamins and they are not doing well, the other vitamins the patient is taking might be the problem.

Start the patient on one-half the normal amount of each suggested nutritional used with this program and only increase every fourth day if they are doing well. The nutritionals used with The Road Back Program will make the other vitamins begin to work and the patient may experience a rapid detox due to the other vitamins. If the patient reacts to the lower introduction amount of the nutritionals used with this program, the only thing left to do is taper the patient off their existing vitamins over a one-month period. Then restart the pre-taper.

I do understand that there are very good and essential vitamins an individual may take, but if the intent is to help the patient off the psychotropic medication, the other vitamins need to wait until the patient is off the medication 45 days.

Titrating Psychoactive Medication:

Have the patient compound his/her medication whenever possible. An exact reduction of the medication each week provides prediction, no guessing, and the highest chance of success.

In the early days of psychoactive drugs, psychiatry did not titrate psychoactive drugs up slowly on patients and the results were catastrophic. Many drugs, other than psychoactive drugs, must be titrated up as well as down before discontinuing.

There seems to be a medical community consensus that psychoactive drugs can be reduced quickly, or patients can abruptly be taken off one psychoactive drug and prescribed another psychoactive drug without an adverse consequence. This is not the case. Even switching a patient from a tablet form of a psychoactive drug to the liquid form of the same psychoactive drug will cause extreme adverse drug reactions.

> Dr. Donald E. McAlpine, psychiatrists at the Mayo Clinic states:
> *"It's important to taper off slowly, extending the taper over several weeks under your physician's direction. When you stop too quickly, you may experience so-called discontinuation symptoms, which can masquerade as relapse."*

The discontinuation process and side effects therein can be confusing to both the patient and physician. Which side effect is coming from the medication, or is it a return of the original symptom?

With a full pre-taper and the person eliminating all, or nearly all, side effects before reducing the medication, rest assured the side effect starting during the taper is due to one of the following:

- **The patient changed something.**
- **The reduction of the medication is too large.**

A change made by the patient can be the most difficult to find. It might be something the patient does not feel is a change.

Years ago I had a person nearly halfway off Paxil. This person experienced no withdrawal side effects tapering the Paxil to that point. When trying to taper off Paxil in the past, the individual had extreme withdrawal side effects after the first reduction attempt and would then need to return to a full dosage.

With no valid explanation, this person began to suffer withdrawal side effect symptoms similar to those earlier. Two weeks passed and I could not find anything the person had changed. Finally, it was mentioned to me by the individual he or she had started an all protein diet, began the diet 3 days before the side effects started.

For this person doing this diet was not a change. He or she would go on this all-protein diet every six months. I give you this example to point out that the change a patient makes may not be so obvious. You may need to dig.

If a patient is keeping a complete Daily Journal these changes can be spotted more quickly and trouble tapering can be avoided.

Use the Suggested Supplements

If you want the standard results with The Road Back Program, use the exact supplements suggested. TRB Health, www.trbhealth.com, (866) 810-3809, has manufactured these supplements to meet our specific requirements for this Program.

GLOSSARY

B.I.D.: Twice a day

ACTH: A hormone produced by the pituitary gland that stimulates the secretion of cortisone and other hormones by the adrenal gland. ACTH is also called adrenocorticotropin, corticotropin.

ADHD: Abbreviation for **A**ttention **D**eficit **H**yperactivity **D**isorder.

ADHD Medication: Medication prescribed for **A**ttention **D**eficit **H**yperactivity **D**isorder. Common medications are Ritalin, Concerta, Adderall and Strattera.

ADRENAL: The adrenal glands (also known as suprarenal glands) are the triangle-shaped endocrine glands that sit on top of the kidneys; their name indicates that position (*ad-*, "near" or "at" + *-renes*, "kidneys"). They are chiefly responsible for regulating the stress response through a chemical reaction. Adrenaline is a "fight or flight" hormone and plays a central role in short-term stress reaction and is released from the adrenal glands when danger threatens or in an emergency. The adrenal gland also produces Cortisol, a vital hormone often referred to as the "stress hormone" since it is involved in the response to stress. It increases blood pressure, blood sugar levels and can suppress the efficiency of the immune system.

AGITATION: Excitement or emotional disturbance.

ALDEHYDE OXIDASE SUBSTRATE: An enzyme pathway the body uses to metabolize substances.

ALKALINE: Something that is alkaline contains an alkali or has a pH value of more than 7. Your body needs a balance between acid and alkali for good health. When pH levels are too low, it means acid is too high in the body. Human bodies are alkaline by design and acid by function. Maintaining proper alkalinity is essential for life, health, and vitality. Simply put, an imbalance of alkalinity creates a condition favorable to the growth of bacteria, yeast and other unwanted organisms. Leading biochemists and medical physiologists have recognized pH (or the acid-alkaline balance) as a key aspect of a balanced and healthy body.

AMINO ACID: Any of a large group of chemical compounds that join together in various ways to form different proteins necessary for life.

AMINE: A chemical compound containing nitrogen, derived from ammonia. The word "amine" derives from "ammonia." Nitrogen is a biologically important colorless, odorless, tasteless gas. It makes up nearly four fifths of the air around the earth, and is found in all living things. Nitrogen, a constituent of protein, is present in all living cells.

ANTIOXIDANT: Any substance that reduces oxidative damage (damage due to oxygen) such as that caused by free radicals. Here's how oxidation works: As oxygen interacts with cells of any type – an apple slice turning brown, or in your body, the cells lining your lungs or in a cut on your skin – oxidation occurs. This produces some type of change in those cells. They may die, such as with rotting fruit. In the case of cut skin, dead cells are replaced in time by fresh, new cells, resulting in a healed cut. Oxidation reaction can produce free radicals, which start chain reactions that damage cells. Free radicals are highly reactive chemicals that attack molecules by capturing electrons and thus modifying chemical structures. Antioxidants terminate these chain reactions by removing free radicals, and inhibit other oxidation reactions by being oxidized themselves. Well-known antioxidants include a number of enzymes and other substances such as vitamin C, vitamin E and beta carotene (which converts to vitamin A) that are capable of counteracting the damaging effects of oxidation.

Free radicals are atoms or molecules with unpaired electrons. These unpaired electrons are usually highly reactive, so radicals are likely to take part in chemical reactions. When free radicals are on the attack, they don't just kill cells to acquire their missing electron. The problem is that free radicals often injure the cell, damaging the DNA, creating the seed for disease. Free radicals trigger a damaging chain reaction. Free radicals are dangerous because they don't damage just one molecule. One free radical can set off a whole chain reaction. When a free radical oxidizes a fatty acid, it changes that fatty acid into a free radical, which then damages another fatty acid. It's a very rapid chain reaction.

ASSIMILATE: To take something in and make it part of oneself; absorb.

AUDIOGENIC SEIZURES: Seizures caused by loud sounds and noises.

AUTONOMIC NERVOUS SYSTEM: That part of the nervous system specifically concerned with the involuntary, seemingly automatic, activities of organs, blood vessels, glands and a variety of other tissues in the body. The autonomic nervous system breaks down into two subordinate systems that work in conjunction with one another: the craniosacral and thoracolumbar. See Craniosacral and Thoracolumbar in this glossary.

BASKET CASE: Someone not doing well emotionally, very nervous and upset.

BASAL METABOLIC RATE: The rate at which the body uses energy when at rest.

BENZODIAZEPINE PROTRACTED WITHDRAWAL: Withdrawal effects from a benzodiazepine that have gone on longer than is normal.

BIOCHEMISTRY: The science dealing with the chemistry of plant and animal life.

BLOOD BRAIN BARRIER (BBB)

A mechanism that controls the passage of substances from the blood into the cerobrospinal fluid (a clear, colorless fluid that bathes the entire surface of the central nervous system and cushions the brain and spinal cord against concussion or violent changes of position) and thus into the brain and spinal cord.

The blood-brain barrier (BBB) lets essential metabolites, such as oxygen and glucose, pass from the blood to the brain and central nervous system (CNS) but blocks most molecules that are more massive. This means that everything from hormones and neurotransmitters to viruses and bacteria are refused access to the brain by the BBB.

Key functions of the BBB are:

- Protecting the brain from "foreign substances" (such as viruses and bacteria) in the blood that could injure the brain.
- Shielding the brain from hormones and neurotransmitters in the rest of the body.
- Maintaining a constant environment (homeostasis) for the brain.

BRAIN ZAPS: "Brain zaps" are a withdrawal symptom experienced during discontinuation (or reduction of dose) of SSRI and SNRI (see definitions of SSRI, SNRI in this glossary) antidepressant drugs. They may also be experienced while the person is actually taking the prescribed medication, and can continue for years after withdrawal from the medication.

The experience is hard to explain if never experienced, but brain zaps basically feel like a sudden "jolt" or an electric shock, followed by a few minutes of light-headedness and disorientation. Physiologically, a "brain zap" is a wave-like electrical pulse that quickly travels across the surface of the brain. Brain zaps occur when withdrawing from SSRI and SNRI antidepressants that have an extremely short elimination half-life; that is, they are more quickly metabolized by the liver and leave the general circulation faster than longer half-life antidepressants. This attribute of abruptness leaves the brain a relatively short time to adapt to a major neuron chemical change when the medication is stopped, and the symptoms may be caused by the brain's attempt to readjust.

Carbohydrate: All carbohydrates are made from sugars. There are a number of different types of sugars but in the body all carbohydrate metabolism converts sugar to glucose, our body's preferred energy source. Glucose is the main sugar present in many foods but some contain different sugars, such as fructose in fruit, lactose in milk, as well as others. Most sugars are digested and absorbed and converted to glucose, some cannot be digested. We call this fiber.

Complex Carbohydrate: ***What are complex carbohydrates?***

Complex carbohydrates or starch are simply sugars bonded together to form a chain. The fiber content causes digestive enzymes to work much harder to access the bonds to break the chain into individual sugars for absorption through the intestines.

For this reason digestion of complex carbohydrates takes longer. The slow absorption of sugars provides us with a steady supply of energy and limits the amount of sugar converted into fat and stored. Some examples of complex carbohydrates are vegetables, whole grain breads, whole grain cereals and legumes.

Simple Carbohydrate: Simple carbohydrates are digested quickly. Many simple carbohydrates contain refined sugars and few essential vitamins and minerals. Examples include fruit juice, milk, honey, white bread, white rice, molasses and sugar.

CATCH 22: An impossible situation because you cannot do one thing until you do another thing, but you cannot do the second thing until you do the first thing.

CELLULAR SUPPORT: Anything that helps and supports the cells at a cellular level.

CHANGE: To make or become different in some way.

CHEMISTRY: The chemistry of an organism are the chemical substances that make it up and the chemical reactions that go on inside it.

CHLOROPHYLL: The green coloring matter in plants; sunlight causes it to change carbon dioxide and water into carbohydrates that are the food of the plant.

CIRCADIAN RYHTHMS: Pertaining to a period of about 24 hours. Applied especially to the rhythmic repetition of certain phenomena in living organisms at about the same time each day. *Circadian rhythms* are regular changes in mental and physical characteristics that occur in the course of a day (*circadian* is Latin for "around a day"). Most circadian rhythms are controlled by the body's biological "clock." Disruption to rhythms usually causes a negative effect. Most travelers have experienced the condition known as jet lag, with its associated symptoms of fatigue, disorientation and insomnia. The rhythm is linked to the light-dark cycle. Light and dark cycles being daytime and night time and how they affect the body.

CIRCUMVENTRICULAR ORGAN: The circumventricular organs are regions of the brain where the blood barrier is weak. These regions allow substances to cross into brain tissue more freely and thereby allow the brain to monitor the makeup of the blood. See also Blood Brain Barrier for more information.

COGENTIN: A drug – **Benztropine mesylate**: **benzatropine mesilate** (marketed as **Cogentin**). It is used in patients to reduce the side effects of antipsychotic treatment.

COLD TURKEY: To stop taking drugs or alcohol without any gradient; stopping quickly or abruptly.

COMPOUND: A substance made up of two or more elements.

COMPOUNDING PHARMACY: Pharmacy is regarded as the science of compounding and dispensing medication; also an establishment used for such purposes. Modern pharmaceutical practice includes the dispensing, identification, selection, and analysis of drugs. **Compounding pharmacies** are on the rise and physicians, medical institutions and patients are realizing more than ever the importance of tailoring an individual's medications to specifically meet their needs. A majority of the pharmacists that are going back to compounding are doing so for the love of the science and interest in the patient's well being. The role of a problem solver opens the door to creativity and genius.

CONJUGATED LINOLEIC ACID (CLA): An unsaturated omega-6 fatty acid.

CONSTANT LEVEL: To maintain a level of a supplement in the body to a degree where it never drops below a certain point.

CONTRA: In opposition to; against.

CONTRASURVIVAL: Opposition to or against survival.

CORTISOL: A hormone produced in the adrenal glands. A vital hormone often referred to as the "stress hormone" as it is involved in the response to stress. It increases blood pressure, blood sugar levels and can reduce the efficiency of the immune system. The synthetic form of cortisol is referred to as hydrocortisone.

CORTISOL LEVELS: Cortisol levels can be too high or too low, each causing problems within the body and hormone balance.

COUMADIN: Coumadin is an anticoagulant (blood thinner) which reduces the formation of blood clots by blocking the synthesis of certain clotting factors. Without these clotting factors, blood clots cannot form. Coumadin is used to prevent heart attacks, strokes, and blood clots in veins and arteries.

CRANIOSACRAL: Pertaining to the craniosacral system. That part of the nervous system concerned mainly with the body's everyday function of excreting waste products. Most active during sleep, slows the heart rate and stimulates the organs of the digestive system because the nerves of this system originate from two regions – the cranial (cranial, meaning of the skull) and sacral (sacral, meaning in the area of the sacrum, a bone at the lower end of the spine forming the back portion of the pelvis).

CUMULATIVE EFFECT: A series of events having a cumulative effect, each event increases the effect.

CYP PATHWAY: An enzyme pathway the body uses to metabolize substances such as drugs. For more information see intermediate metabolizer.

CYP 2D6: An enzyme pathway the body uses to metabolize substances such as drugs.

CYP 2C19: An enzyme pathway the body uses to metabolize substances such as drugs.

CYP 3A: An enzyme pathway the body uses to metabolize substances such as drugs.

DAILY JOURNAL: An account on which you write your daily activities.

DETOXIFICATION: The act of removing all the poisonous or harmful substances from something.

DEVIATION: Doing something that is different from what people consider normal or acceptable.

DISCONTINUATION SYMPTOMS: The side effects or reactions people get when stopping a drug.

DHA: (Docosahexanoic) Docosahexaenoic acid commonly known as **DHA**; it is an omega-3 essential fatty acid. **Essential fatty acids**, or EFAs, are fatty acids that cannot be constructed within an organism from other components (generally all references are to humans) by any known chemical pathways; and therefore must be obtained from diet. The term refers to those involved in biological processes, and not fatty acids which may just play a role as fuel.

DNA: Deoxyribonucleic acid (DNA) DNA contains the genetic information for the reproduction of life. DNA is a nucleic acid that contains the genetic instructions used in the development and functioning of all known living organisms and some viruses. The main role of DNA molecules is the long-term storage of information. DNA is often compared to a set of blueprints or a recipe, since it contains the instructions needed to construct other components of cells, such as proteins. The DNA segments that carry this genetic information are called genes, but other DNA sequences have structural purposes, or are involved in regulating the use of this genetic information.

DOUBLE-BLIND RANDOMIZED CONTROLLED TRIALS: Double-blind: Term used to describe a study in which both the investigator or the participant are blind to (unaware of) the nature of the treatment the participant is receiving. Double-blind trials are thought to produce objective results, since the expectations of the researcher and the participant about the experimental treatment such as a drug do not affect the outcome.

DRUG/DRUG INTERACTION: The interaction between one drug and another drug and the effect created.

DRUG INSERTS: Material, called package inserts, providing information on the usage and risks of medications – including warnings, side effects, contraindications and interactions with other drugs. The FDA says it is concerned that the old format, plus information overload, mean that some of the information may not be getting through to doctors and consumers, resulting in thousands of "preventable adverse events" every year.

DRUG/SUPPLEMENT INTERACTIONS: The interaction between a drug and a supplement and the effect created.

ELECTROLYTE BALANCE: Electrolyte is a "medical/scientific" term for salts, specifically ions. The term electrolyte means this ion is electrically-charged and moves to either a negative or positive electrode.

Electrolytes are important because they are what your cells (especially nerve, heart, muscle) use to maintain voltages across cell membranes and carry electrical impulses (nerve impulses, muscle contractions) across themselves and to other cells. Your kidneys work to keep the electrolyte concentrations in your blood constant despite changes in your body. For example, when you exercise heavily, you lose electrolytes in your sweat, particularly sodium and potassium. These electrolytes must be replaced to keep body fluids electrolyte concentrations constant.

Electrolyte levels can become too low or too high which can happen when the amount of water in your body changes. Causes include some medicines, vomiting, diarrhea, sweating or kidney problems. Problems most often occur with levels of sodium, potassium or calcium.

ELECTRONICS: The branch of physics that deals with electrons in motion.

EMOTIONAL: Concerned with feelings and emotions.

ENDOCRINE: The system of glands that produce hormones http://en.wikipedia.org/wiki/Image:Illu_endocrine_system.jpg. Endocrine glands release hormones (chemical messengers) into the bloodstream to be transported to various organs and tissues throughout the body.

EPA: Eicosapentaenoic acid (EPA) is an omega-3 fatty acid.

ESTROGEN: A female hormone produced primarily in the ovaries. Some estrogens are also produced in smaller amounts by other tissues such as the liver, adrenal glands and the breasts. These secondary sources of estrogen are especially important in postmenopausal women. Estrogen deficiency can lead to osteoporosis (a condition in which bones lose calcium and become more likely to break).

EXACERBATE: If something exacerbates a problem, it makes it worse.

EXTENSIVE METABOLIZER: Approximately half of all Americans have genetic defects that affect how they process drugs. There are four different types of metabolizers. We all fall into one of these categories for the variable pathways in Cytochrome P450 (this Cytochrome is responsible for creating the enzymes that process chemicals of all kinds through our bodies.) The easiest way to understand this is to picture a two lane highway. If you are the first type which is the **norm**, you would be an **EXTENSIVE metabolizer**. Both lanes of the highway are open and moving. Medications prescribed in normal doses will be metabolized by your body.

EXTREME: To the greatest degree; very great; excessive. 2. farthest away 3. far from what is usual.

FEEDBACK LOOP: Feedback is both a mechanism, process and signal that is looped back to control a system within itself. This loop is called the feedback loop. A control system usually has input and output to the system; when the output of the system is fed back into the system as part of its input, it is called the "feedback." In a feedback loop, increased amounts of a substance – for example, a hormone – inhibit the release of more of that substance, while decreased amounts of the substance stimulate the release of more of that substance.

FLAT LINED: A **flatline** is an electrical time sequence measurement that shows no activity and therefore when represented, shows a flat line instead of a moving one. This term almost always refers to either a flatlined electrocardiogram, where the heart shows no electrical activity, or to a flat electroencephalogram, in which the brain shows no electrical activity (brain death). Both of these specific cases are involved in various definitions of death. Some consider one who has flatlined to have been clinically dead, regardless of their eventual resuscitation or lack thereof, whereas others insist that one is alive until the moment of brain death. Term mostly used in the medical industry when a person's pulse has stopped, indicating a flat line on the heart monitor. **Flat-lined** in this book is used figuratively to mean having no emotion or feeling.

FRAY: fight, battle, or skirmish; a noisy quarrel or brawl.

FREE-RADICAL: Atoms or molecules with unpaired electrons. These unpaired electrons are usually highly reactive, so radicals are likely to take part in chemical reactions. When free radicals are on the attack, they don't just kill cells to acquire their missing molecule. Free radicals often injure the cell, damaging the DNA, which creates the seed for disease. Free radicals trigger a damaging chain reaction. Free radicals are dangerous because they don't just damage one molecule. One free radical can set off a whole chain reaction. When a free radical oxidizes a fatty acid, it changes that fatty acid into a free radical, which then damages another fatty acid. It's a very rapid chain reaction.

FMO: An enzyme pathway the body uses to metabolize substances such as drugs.

GLUCOSE (Glc): A monosaccharide (or simple sugar) also known as **grape sugar**; an important carbohydrate. The living cell uses it as a source of energy. Glucose is one of the main products of photosynthesis **(Photosynthesis** is the conversion of light energy into chemical energy by living organisms) and starts cellular respiration (**Cellular respiration** – the reactions and processes that take place in a cell or across the cell membrane to release energy from nutrients and then release waste products). The name comes from the Greek word *glykys* (γλυκύς), meaning "sweet", plus the suffix "-ose" denoting a sugar.

Glucaronic acid: An acid formed by the oxidation of glucose, found combined with other products of metabolism in the blood and urine.

GLUCURONIDATION: A phase II detoxification pathway occurring in the liver in which glucuronic acid is joined together with toxins. It effectively detoxifies the majority of commonly prescribed drugs. Thus, glucuronidation represents a major means of converting most drugs, steroids and many toxic substances to metabolites that can then be excreted into the urine or bile.

GLUTATHIONE (GSH): A naturally occurring protein that protects every cell, tissue and organ from toxic free radicals and disease. It is a **tripeptide** of three amino acids - glycine, glutamate (glutamic acid) and cysteine (**tripeptide** is a **peptide** consisting of three amino acids). These **precursors** (**precursors** are substances from which something else is formed) are necessary for the manufacture of glutathione within the cells. Glutathione has been called the "master antioxidant" and regulates the actions of lesser antioxidants such as vitamin C and vitamin E within the body.

Peptide: A molecule consisting of 2 or more amino acids. Peptides are smaller than proteins, which are also chains of amino acids. Molecules small enough to be synthesized from the constituent amino acids are, by convention, called peptides rather than proteins.

GUT: The stomach or belly.

HALF-LIFE: If you draw a graph of drug levels in the blood, you will see that they rise quickly after a dose is taken, then fall off over time until the next dose. When this blood level drops by 50% that would be half-life.

HAMILTON ANXIETY SCORE: The Hamilton Anxiety Scale (HAS or HAMA) is a 14-item test measuring the severity of anxiety symptoms. It is also sometimes called the Hamilton Anxiety Rating Scale (HARS). The score would be the result of the test with a number value.

HAVING YOUR CAKE AND EATING IT TOO: To wish to **have one's cake and eat it too** or simply **have one's cake and eat it** (sometimes **eat one's cake and have it too**) is to want more than one can handle or deserve, or to try to have two incompatible things.

HAY FEVER: Allergy caused by the pollen of ragweed, trees, grasses and other plants, characterized by itching, and running eyes and nose and fits of sneezing.

HEAVY METAL CHELATING: Introduction of certain substances into the body so that they will chelate, and then remove, foreign substances such as lead, cadmium, arsenic and other heavy metals. Chelation therapy can also be used to reduce or remove calcium-based plaque from the linings of the blood vessels, easing the flow of blood to vital organs and tissues. *Chelation* is a chemical process by which a larger molecule or group of molecules surround or enclose a mineral atom. One source defines "heavy metal" as common transition metals, such as copper, lead and zinc. These metals are a cause of environmental pollution (heavy-metal pollution) from a number of sources, including lead in petrol, industrial waste, and leaching of metal ions from the soil into lakes and rivers by acid rain.

HEPATIC 3A: Hepatic means having to do with the liver, *see CYP 3A*.

HOMEOSTASIS: The tendency to maintain, or the maintenance of, normal, internal stability in an organism by coordinated responses of the organ systems that automatically readjust for environmental changes.

HORMONES: Essential substances produced by the endocrine glands that regulate bodily functions; a regulatory substance produced in an organism and transported in tissue fluids such as blood to stimulate cells or tissues into action. **Hormones** are chemicals released by cells that affect cells in other parts of the body. Only a small amount of hormone is required to alter cell metabolism. Also act as chemical messengers that transport a signal from one cell to another.

GLOSSARY

HPA: The Hypothalamus-Pituitary-Adrenal (HPA) axis is one of the key parts of the human endocrine system. As its name suggests, it comprises three endocrine glands, the hypothalamus, the (anterior) pituitary, and the adrenal gland cortex.

Hypothalamic-Pituitary-Adrenal Axis

What is the HPA axis?

The hypothalamus is the control center for most of body's hormonal systems. Follow figure 1 as I explain this. Cells in the hypothalamus produce hormone corticotrophin-releasing factor (CRF) in humans in response to most any type of stress – physical or psychological.

The hypothalamus secretes CRF, which in turn binds to specific receptors on pituitary cells, which produce adrenocorticotropic hormone (ACTH). ACTH is then transported to its target the adrenal gland. The adrenal gland then stimulates the production of adrenal hormones which increase the secretion of cortisol.

The release of cortisol initiates a series of metabolic effects aimed at alleviating the harmful effects of stress through negative feedback to both the hypothalamus and the anterior pituitary, which decreases the concentration of ACTH and cortisol in the blood once the state of stress subsides.

HYPER: A prefix meaning over, more than normal, too much.

HYPERAGGRESSION: Too much aggression.

HYPERKINESIAS: An abnormal increase in muscular activity, hyperactivity, especially in children.

HYPER METABOLIZER: Someone that metabolizes too much.

HYPERTHERMIA: Unusually high body temperature.

HYPOTHALAMUS: The **hypothalamus** links the nervous system to the endocrine system via the pituitary gland. The hypothalamus is located below the thalamus, just above the brain stem. It is also responsible for the motivation of what has been called the "Four F's"(feeding, fighting, fleeing and sexual reproduction (fertility).

The hypothalamus controls body temperature, hunger, thirst, fatigue, anger and circadian cycles.

HYPOTHALAMUS-PITUITARY-ADRENAL AXIS: See HPA

IMMUNE SYSTEM: A complex system that depends on the interaction of many different organs, cells, and proteins. Its chief function is to identify and eliminate foreign substances such as harmful bacteria that have invaded the body. The liver, spleen, thymus, bone marrow and lymphatic system all play vital roles in the proper functioning

(Picture following.)

INDUCER: An inducer is a molecule that starts gene expression. **Gene expression** is the process by which inheritable information from a gene, such as the DNA sequence, is made into a functional gene product, such as protein.

INFLAMMATORY: Inflammation of the body. Inflammation is a localized physical condition with heat, swelling, redness and usually pain especially as a reaction to injury or infection.

INHIBITOR DRUGS: A drug which restrains or retards physiological, chemical, or enzymatic action.

INSOMNIA: Inability to sleep; abnormal wakefulness.

INSULIN: A protein hormone formed in the pancreas and secreted into the blood, where it regulates carbohydrate (sugar) metabolism.

INTERLUEKIN: Interleukins are a group of cytokines (secreted signaling molecules) that were first seen to be expressed by white blood cells (leukocytes, hence the *-leukin*) as a means of communication (*inter-*). Interleukins are produced by a wide variety of bodily cells. The function of the immune system depends in a large part on *interleukins*.

INTERLUEKIN 6 (IL-6): Made by the body, interluekin-6 (IL-6) is a type of protein that helps regulate the immune system. It can also serve as a liver cell growth factor. IL-6 is needed in the body. However, too much IL-6 will promote inflammation and has been shown to be a direct link to chronic depression.

INTERLUEKIN 2(IL-2): Interleukin-2 is a type of protein found in the immune system that is instrumental to the body's natural response to microbial infection and in discriminating between foreign and self.

INTERMEDIATE METABOLIZER: Of all the clinical factors that alter a person's response to drugs (age, sex, weight, general health and liver function, etc.) genetic factors are the most important. This information becomes crucial when you consider that adverse reactions to prescription drugs are killing about 106,000 Americans each year – roughly three times as many killed by automobiles.

Approximately half of all Americans have genetic defects that affect how they process drugs. There are four different types of metabolizers. We all fall into one of these categories for the variable pathways in Cytochrome P450 (this Cytochrome is responsible for creating the enzymes that process chemicals of all kinds through our bodies).

The easiest way to understand this is to picture a two-lane highway.

If you are the second type, you would be an INTERMEDIATE metabolizer. This means that one lane of that highway is open and moving and the other lane is not, causing you to metabolize the medications more slowly. In this case you will need a lower dosage, and there is a chance of medications building up in your system causing adverse effects. Monitoring medications is especially important if you are in this category.

INTESTINAL 3A: An enzyme pathway the body uses to metabolize substances such as drugs.

INTRACELLULAR: Intra means occurring within; intracellular means occurring within the cell.

IONIC BALANCE: (or electrolyte balance) Balance of fluid in the body fluid compartments; total body water, blood volume, maintained by processes in the body that regulate the intake and excretion of water and electrolytes, particularly sodium and potassium.

ION: an atom or group of atoms having a charge of positive or negative electricity.

IONIC CALCIUM: Ionic means pertaining to ions. Ionic calcium would be calcium that is electrically charged. The type of calcium that fizzes when put it in water. The body breaks down calcium and will turn it ionic through the process of absorption. Using ionic calcium bypasses this action of the body.

IRRITABLE BOWEL SYNDROME (IBS): irritable bowel syndrome (IBS) is a bowel disorder characterized by mild to severe abdominal pain, discomfort, bloating and alteration of bowel habits. In some cases, the symptoms are relieved by bowel movements.

JOURNAL: A daily record of events.

KRILL: Small, shrimp-like fish that swim in the sea.

LECITHIN: A fatlike substance produced daily by the liver if the diet is adequate. Lecithin is needed by every cell in the body and is a key building block of cell membranes. Without lecithin, cells would harden. Lecithin protects cells from oxidation and largely comprises the protective sheaths surrounding the brain. It is composed mostly of B vitamins, phosphoric acid, choline, linoleic acid and inositol.

LIFE: The quality that distinguishes a vital and functional being from a dead body or inanimate matter (Webster's Dictionary).

LIGHT/DARK CYCLES: see Circadian Rhythms.

LIMBIC SYSTEM: The **limbic system** is a term for a set of brain structures that support a variety of functions including emotion, behavior and long term memory. The structures of the brain described by the limbic system are closely associated with the sense of smell structures. The term "limbic" comes from Latin *limbus*, meaning "border" or "belt."

LYMPH SYSTEM: Part of the immune system with lymph nodes and tissues. The role of tissue fluid is to deliver the groceries to the cells. The role of lymph is to take out the trash that is left behind and dispose of it.

As lymph continues to circulate between the cells it collects waste products that were left behind including dead blood cells, pathogens and cancer cells. This clear fluid also becomes protein-rich as it absorbs dissolved protein from between the cells.

MACROECONOMICS: Macro is added to words that refer to things that are large in size or broad in scope. Macroeconomics means relating to the major, general features of a country's economy such as unemployment and interest rates.

MAJOR CHANGE: A change that is significant.

MAJOR IMPROVEMENTS: An improvement that is significant.

MAJOR POSITIVE CHANGE: A change that is significant and for the better.

MEDICATION INDUCED SIDE EFFECTS: Side effects caused by medication.

MELATONIN: A hormone produced by the pineal gland, intimately involved in regulating the sleeping and waking cycles among other processes. Melatonin supplements are sometimes used by people to handle chronic insomnia. Always see your doctor before taking melatonin, as it is not always recommended for sleep problems.

MEMBRANE: A thin layer of tissue which covers a surface or divides a space or organ.

METABOLIZING ROUTE: An enzyme pathway used to metabolize something in the body.

MINERALS: An inorganic substance required by the body in small quantities.

MUCUS LINING: The moist lining of a body cavity or structure, such as the mouth or nose.

NARCOTICS: Drugs such as opium or heroin which induce sleep and inhibit pain sensation.

NATUROPATH: A health care practitioner that uses diet, herbs and other natural methods and substances to cure illness. The goal is to produce a healthy body state by stimulating innate defenses and without the use of drugs.

NEURAL TISSUE: Neural means pertaining to a nerve or to the nerves. Neural tissue is specialized for the conduction of electrical impulses that convey information or instructions from one region of the body to another. About 98% of neural tissue is concentrated in the brain and spinal cord, the control centers for the nervous system.

NORMAL METABOLIZER: See extensive metabolizer.

NUCLEI: Plural of nucleus

NUCLEUS: The small mass at the center of most living cells.

NUTRIENT: A substance that is needed by the body to maintain life and health.

OLFACTORY SYSTEM: The sensory system used for the sense of smell

OPIATES: A remedy containing or derived from opium; also any drug that induces sleep.

OSMORECEPTER: A specialized sensory nerve ending sensitive to stimulation giving rise to the sensation of odors.

OVLT: The **organum vasculosum of the lamina terminalis (OVLT)** is one of the **circumventricular organs** of the brain .**Circumventricular organs** are so named because they are positioned at distinct sites around the margin of the **ventricular system** of the brain. The **ventricular system** is a set of structures in the brain continuous with the central canal of the spinal cord. See **Circumventricular organs.**

PARASYMPATHETIC SYSTEM: The part of the autonomic nervous system originating in the brain stem and the lower part of the spinal cord that, in general, inhibits or opposes the physiological effects of the **sympathetic nervous system**, as in tending to stimulate digestive secretions, slow the heart, constrict the pupils and dilate blood vessels. The **Sympathetic Nervous System** is a branch of the autonomic nervous system. It is always active and becomes more active during times of stress. Its actions during the stress response are the opposite of the parasympathetic system which is to expand pupils, accelerate heart beat, inhibit digestion and relax the bladder. The **autonomic nervous system** acts as a control system, maintaining balance in the body.

PATHWAY: A particular course of action; *medical;* The sequence of enzymatic steps in the process by which something is metabolized in the body.

P450 (CYP) ENZYMES: An enzyme pathway the body uses to metabolize substances such as drugs.

P-gp: An enzyme pathway the body uses to metabolize substances.

PHASE II LIVER DETOX GENES: To be effective a detox diet must do a few things. First and foremost, a detox diet must increase the phase II of the liver. The liver uses two phases to breakdown chemical toxins.

Phase I: At the end of phase I the liver has accumulated the toxins but they are now in their raw state. This is the stage where your body is the most exposed to toxins. The liver is now holding the toxins in their most toxic state.

Phase II: The liver passes the toxins over to the phase II process. If the phase II process is not functioning properly, the toxins will not be removed and the raw toxins may be dumped back into the body. Phase II is where the toxins are carried out of the body. It is vital during a liver detox that phase II is fully activated. It is also during phase II that glutathione comes into play. Glutathione being activated is every bit as vital during the phase II process of a detox.

There are probably as many viewpoints about how to detox as there are products being sold to handle a detox. However, it does come down to only two actions within the liver, phase I and phase II, the breaking down of toxins and moving them out of the body.

There are 3 genes that regulate the phase II of the liver. The gene names are: **GSTM1, GSTT1, and GSTP1**. The G stands for Glutathione. At least 50% of the population will have 1 or more of these genes with a variation. The people with a variation in their detox genes will have a more difficult time removing toxins and will need help making glutathione within the liver.

PHOSPHOLIPIDS: Phospholipids are the building blocks of *every cell* in the human body and that includes nerve cells, tissues, blood vessels and skin. Phospholipids protect the body from free-radical attack and toxic injury.

PHYSICAL STRESSORS: Physical Stressors result from internal physical symptoms, such as headaches, stomach problems, etc. and external physical stressors, such as heat, cold, excessive noise, etc.

GLOSSARY

PLATELETS: A circular oval disk found in the blood which is concerned with coagulation (clotting the blood to stop a wound's bleeding).

POOR METABOLIZER: Approximately half of all Americans have genetic defects that affect how they process these drugs. There are four different types of metabolizers. We all fall into one of these categories for the variable pathways in Cytochrome P450 (this Cytochrome is responsible for creating the enzymes that process chemicals of all kinds through our bodies). The easiest way to understand this is to picture a two lane highway.

If you are the first type which is the norm, you would be an EXTENSIVE metabolizer. Both lanes of the highway are open and moving. Medications prescribed in normal doses will be metabolized by your body.

The third type is a **POOR metabolizer**. In this case both lanes of the highway would be stopped. There is a possibility that alternate routes can be found, but this type of metabolization is potentially very dangerous, as there is a great chance for the medication to build up in your system making you very sick, or even killing you.

For example, a poor metabolizer of phenytoin, a common anti-seizure medication would not be able to process the drug and would actually have an increased rather than decreased risk of seizure if prescribed this drug.

POSTREMA: The **area postrema** is a part of the brain that controls vomiting. The area postrema detects toxins in the blood and acts as a vomit inducing center.

POST TRAUMATIC STRESS DISORDER (PTSD): An anxiety disorder that can develop after exposure to one or more terrifying events in which grave physical harm occurred or was threatened. It is a severe and ongoing emotional reaction to an extreme psychological trauma. The stressor may involve someone's actual death or a threat to the patient's or someone else's life, serious physical injury, or threat to physical and/or psychological integrity, to a degree with which usual psychological defenses cannot cope.

In some cases it can also be from profound psychological and emotional trauma, apart from any actual physical harm. Often, however, the two are combined.

PRE-TAPER: Pre means before and taper means to gradually reduce in size or amount. Pre-taper is something you do before a taper.

PROPRIETARY: Owned by a person or company, as under a patent, trademark or copyright.

PROSURVIVAL: Pro means to support, be in favor of; for. Prosurvival means to support or be in favor or survival.

PROTOCOL: Is a course of treatment for someone who is ill or has an addiction.

PROTRACTED: When something has gone on longer than is usual or expected, usually something unpleasant.

PSYCHOACTIVE MEDICATIONS: A psychoactive drug or **psychotropic substance** is a chemical substance that acts primarily upon the central nervous system where it alters brain function, resulting in temporary changes in perception, mood, consciousness and behavior.

PSYCHOSIS: A psychiatric term for a mental state often described as involving a "loss of contact with reality." People suffering from it are said to be **psychotic.**

People experiencing psychosis may report hallucinations or delusional beliefs, and may exhibit personality changes and disorganized thinking. This may be accompanied by unusual or bizarre behavior, as well as difficulty with social interaction and impairment in carrying out the activities of daily living.

A wide variety of central nervous system diseases, from both external toxins and from internal physiologic illness, can produce symptoms of psychosis.

PSYCHOTROPIC: Having an altering effect on perception, emotion, or behavior. Used especially of a drug.

PHYSIOLOGY: The scientific study of how human and animal bodies function and how plants function.

PREBIOTICS: Indigestible carbohydrates that stimulate the growth and activity of beneficial bacteria (probiotics) of the intestinal flora.

PROBIOTICS: Your body contains billions of bacteria and other microorganisms. The term "probiotics" refers to dietary supplements or foods that contain beneficial or "good" bacteria similar to those normally found in the body. Although you don't need probiotics to be healthy, these microorganisms may provide some of the same health benefits that the bacteria already existing in your body do – such as assisting with digestion and helping protect against harmful bacteria.

PTSD: See **P**ost **T**raumatic **S**tress **D**isorder.

QUANDARY: State of being uncertain; dilemma.

REACH: 1. To extend out. 2. To touch or to seize 3. To communicate with.

RECEPTORS: Nerve endings in the body which react to changes and stimuli and make your body respond in a particular way.

RELAPSE: To fall back into an earlier condition.

RENAL EXTRACTION: The term "renal" refers to the kidneys. Testing waste coming out of the body to see how much of a drug or substance was left in the body and what is not.

RETICULAR FORMATION: The **reticular formation** is a part of the brain that is involved in actions such as waking/sleeping cycle and lying down. It is essential for governing some of the basic functions of higher organisms, and is one of the oldest portions of the brain. A network of nerve fibers and cells in parts of the brainstem, important in regulating consciousness or wakefulness.

ROLLED A SEVEN: To get lucky by chance.

SCENARIO: A likely or possible **scenario** means the way in which a situation may or has developed.

SCORED: "Tablets are scored." **Scoring** a surface with something sharp means cutting or scratch a line in it.

SELF MEDICATE: Self-medication is the use of drugs to treat a perceived or real malady. Over-the-counter drugs are a form of self medication. The buyer diagnoses his/her own illness and buys a specific drug to treat it. The World Self-Medication Industry (WSMI) defines self-medication as *the treatment of common health problems with medicines especially designed and labeled for use without medical supervision and approved as safe and effective for such use.* A person may also self-medicate by taking more or less than the recommended dose of a drug.

SET-POINT: An arbitrary point for each individual and within each individual's body. The various hormones and endocrine etc. have their own point of reference that is ideal for that body.

7 RATING: A rating on how you are doing kept in your journal on The Road Back Program. A 7-10 rating is a rating that you are doing well. You rate how you feel, your energy, appetite, mood and exercise.

SHORT CHAIN FATTY ACIDS: Fatty acids taken up directly to the portal vein (a large vein that carries blood from the digestive tract to the liver) during digestion of fat. Produced when dietary fiber is fermented in the colon.

SIDE EFFECTS: Problems that occur when treatment goes beyond the desired effect or problems that occur in addition to the desired therapeutic effect.

Example – A hemorrhage from the use of too much anticoagulant (such as heparin) is a side effect caused by treatment going beyond the desired effect.

Example – Common side effects of cancer treatment including fatigue, nausea, vomiting, decreased blood cell counts, hair loss and mouth sores. They occur in addition to the desired therapeutic effect.

Drug manufacturers are required to list all known side effects of their products.

SLEEP MEDICATION: A drug that puts you to sleep.

SLOW METABOLIZER: See poor metabolizer.

SNRI: Serotonin-norepinephrine reuptake inhibitors (SNRIs) are a class of antidepressant used in the treatment of major depression and other mood disorders. Also sometimes used to treat anxiety disorders, obsessive-compulsive disorder, attention deficit hyperactivity disorder (ADHD) and chronic neuropathic pain.

SOLUBLE: Can be dissolved in a liquid.

SSRI: **Selective serotonin reuptake inhibitors (SSRIs)** are a class of antidepressants used in the treatment of depression, anxiety disorders and some personality disorders. They are also used in treating premature ejaculation problems as well as some cases of insomnia

STAGE 1 DETOXIFICATION: You have completed Stage 1 Detoxification by coming off the medications.

STAGE 2 DETOXIFICATION: The process of removing the remaining toxins from the body. There will be drug toxins remaining in the body as well other toxins picked up by living on planet earth.

STAGE 2 SLEEP: In this stage (the beginning of "true" sleep) the person's electroencephalogram (EEG) will show distinctive wave forms. About 50% of sleep time is stage 2 sleep. **Electroencephalography** (EEG) is the measurement of electrical activity produced by the brain.

STEADY STATE: A constant level or a level of action that allows a balance between two or more substances.

SUPER FOODS: Highly nutritious supplements considered to have a complete array of all vitamins, minerals and amino acids the human body may need.

SUPRACHIASMATIC NUCLEUS: The **suprachiasmatic nucleus** (SCN) is a region of the brain (located in the hypothalamus) responsible for controlling from within the body circadian rhythms (see circadian rhythms). The neuronal and hormonal activities it generates regulate many different body functions over a 24-hour period. The suprachiasmatic nucleus of the hypothalamus (SCN) contains a master circadian pacemaker. Biological rhythms are synchronized by light and darkness.

SYMPATHETIC SYSTEM: Sympathetic Nervous System is a branch of the autonomic nervous system. Always active, it becomes more active during times of stress. Its actions during the stress response are the opposite of the parasympathetic system which is to expand pupils, accelerate heart beat, inhibit digestion and relax the bladder. The **autonomic nervous system** acts as a control system, maintaining balance in the body.

SYSTEMATIC: Done according to a fixed plan, in a thorough and efficient way.

SYSTEMIC: Having to do with the body as a whole. Systemic chemicals or drugs are absorbed into the whole of the body rather than being applied to one area.

TAPER: To gradually become reduced in amount, number or size until it is greatly reduced.

TESTOSTERONE: A white crystalline steroid hormone, produced primarily in the testes and responsible for the development and maintenance of male secondary sex characteristics. Also produced synthetically for use in medical treatments.

THERMORECEPTOR: Sensory receptor that responds to heat and cold.

Sensory receptors account for our ability to see, hear, taste and smell, and to sense touch, pain, temperature and body position. They also provide the unconscious ability of the body to detect changes in blood volume, blood pressure, and the levels of salts, gases and nutrients in the blood.

These specialized cells are exquisitely adapted for the detection of particular physical or chemical events outside the cell. They are connected to nerve cells, or are themselves nerve cells.

THORACOLUMBAR: Pertaining to the thoracolumbar system. That part of the nervous system mainly concerned with preparing the body for action particularly during times of stress, excitement or fear. It acts to stimulate such functions as heart rate, sweating and blood flow to the muscles while at the same time decreasing the activity of the digestive system. Called the thoracolumbar system because the nerves of this system originate from two regions of the spine: the thoracic (meaning of the thorax, that area of the body between the neck and the abdomen; chest) and the lumbar (meaning of the lower part of the back below the thorax).

THYROID: A small gland, normally weighing less than one ounce, located in the front of the neck. Made up of two halves, called lobes, that lie along the windpipe (trachea) joined together by a narrow band of thyroid tissue, known as the isthmus.

The thyroid is situated just below the "Adams apple" or larynx. During development (inside the womb) the thyroid gland originates in the back of the tongue, but normally migrates to the front of the neck before birth. Very rarely it fails to migrate properly and is located high in the neck or even in the back of the tongue (lingual thyroid). Also very rarely at other times it may migrate too far and ends up in the chest.

The thyroid gland takes iodine, found in many foods, and converts it into thyroid hormones: thyroxine (T4) and triiodothyronine (T3). Thyroid cells are the only cells in the body which can absorb iodine. These cells combine iodine and the amino acid **tyrosine** to make T3 and T4. T3 and T4 are then released into the blood stream and transported throughout the body where they control metabolism (conversion of oxygen and calories to energy). **Every cell in the body depends upon thyroid hormones for regulation of metabolism.** The normal thyroid gland produces about 80% T4 and about 20% T3. However, T3 possesses about four times the hormone "strength" as T4.

The pituitary gland (a small gland the size of a peanut at the base of the brain) **controls the thyroid gland.** When the thyroid hormones levels (T3 & T4) drop too low, the pituitary gland produces **Thyroid Stimulating Hormone (TSH)** which stimulates the thyroid gland to produce more hormones. Under the influence of TSH, the thyroid will manufacture and secrete T3 and T4 thereby raising their levels in the blood. The pituitary senses this and responds by decreasing TSH production. Imagine the thyroid gland as a furnace and the pituitary gland as the thermostat. Thyroid hormones are like heat. When the heat hits a certain level, the turns thermostat turns off. As the room cools (the thyroid hormone levels drop), the thermostat turns back on (TSH increases) and the furnace produces more heat (thyroid hormones).

The pituitary gland itself is regulated by another gland, known as the hypothalamus. The hypothalamus is part of the brain and produces **TSH Releasing Hormone (TRH)** which tells the pituitary gland to stimulate the thyroid gland (release TSH). One might imagine the hypothalamus as the person who regulates the thermostat since it tells the pituitary gland at what level the thyroid should be set.

The thyroid gland, a part of the endocrine (hormone) system, plays a major role in regulating the body's metabolism.

Hypothyroidism is a decreased activity of the thyroid gland which may affect all body functions. The metabolism rate slows causing mental and physical sluggishness. Hypothyroidism can be caused by a thyroid problem (primary), or by the malfunction of the pituitary gland or hypothalamus (secondary).

THYROID-STIMULATING HORMONE: When the level of thyroid hormones (T3 & T4) drops too low, the pituitary gland produces **Thyroid Stimulating Hormone (TSH)** which stimulates the thyroid gland to produce more hormones.

TITRATING MEDICATION: Continuously measure and adjust the balance of a drug dosage.

TRAUMATIC STRESS: One or more terrifying events in which grave physical harm occurred or was threatened. This stressor may involve serious physical injury, someone's actual death or a threat to the patient's or someone else's life.

TREPIDATION: A term meaning, in general, the fear or trembling. (from Lat. *trepidus*, "anxious")

TSH: See Thyroid Stimulating Hormone.

2A6: An enzyme pathway the body uses to metabolize substances.

2B6: An enzyme pathway the body uses to metabolize substances.

2E1: An enzyme pathway the body uses to metabolize substances.

UGT1A1: This gene encodes an enzyme of a pathway that transforms small molecules, such as steroids, excreted bile, hormones and drugs into water-soluble, excretable substances that have been metabolized.

Lack of UGT1A1 in a newborn's liver is the major cause of jaundice. This jaundice is generally caused by the natural breakdown of fetal blood cells which produces bilirubin that cannot be cleared if UGT1A1 is expressed at low levels or is absent. This type of jaundice can remedied by UV light exposure.

UGT1A3, UGT1A4, UGTIA6, UTGIA9: Human genes used in metabolizing substances in the body. Each gene encodes an enzyme of a pathway that transforms small molecules, such as steroids, excreted bile, hormones and drugs, into water-soluble, excretable substances that have been metabolized.

UGT2B15: A human gene. The UGTs are of major importance in the joining and subsequent elimination of potentially toxic compounds.

UGT2B7: (UDP-Glucuronosyltransferase-2B7) is a phase II metabolism enzyme found to be active in the liver, kidneys, cells of the lower gastrointestinal tract and has also been reported in the brain.**UGT2B7** is the major enzyme for the metabolism of morphine.

UNDENATURED: Not having its nature or structure changed; in a natural state not changed in any way.

VAGUS: The vagus nerve, or cranial nerve X, is a part of the autonomic nervous system, which controls functions of the body not under voluntary control, such as heart rate and digestion. The **vagus nerve** is the only nerve that starts in the brain stem and extends down below the head, to the neck, chest and abdomen.

The medieval Latin word vagus means literally "wandering" (the words vagrant, *vagabond*, and vague come from the same root).

VASOCONSTRICTION: The narrowing of the blood vessels resulting from contraction of the vessel muscular walls. When blood vessels constrict, the flow of blood is restricted or slowed. Factors causing vasoconstriction are called **vasoconstrictor**, also **vasopressors** or simply **pressors**. Vasoconstriction usually results in increased blood pressure. Vasoconstriction may be slight or severe. Vasoconstriction in the penis can disable males from maintaining an erection (erectile dysfunction). It may result from disease, medication or psychological conditions. Medications that cause vasoconstriction include antihistamines, decongestants, methylphenidate (commonly used for ADHD), cough and cold combinations, pseudoephedrine and caffeine.

VASOPRESSIN SECRETION: Arginine vasopressin (AVP), also known as **vasopressin**, **argipressin** or **antidiuretic hormone (ADH)** A hormone found in most mammals, including humans. Primarily increases water re-absorption in the kidneys.

VITAMIN: One of approximately fifteen organic substances essential in small quantities for life and health. Most vitamins cannot be manufactured by the body thus need to be supplied in the diet.

WHEY ISOLATE PROTEIN: Isolate means to separate (a substance) in pure form from a combined mixture. **Whey** is the watery part of milk that separates from the curd, as in the process of making cheese. **What is whey protein?** A pure, natural, high quality protein from cow's milk; a rich source of the essential amino acids needed on a daily basis by the body. Its purest form, whey protein isolate, contains little to no fat, lactose or cholesterol.

WITHDRAWAL SIDE EFFECTS: The reactions that occur in your body when you withdraw the use of a drug.

WILLY NILLY: 1. Whether desired or not: *After her boss fell sick, she willy-nilly found herself directing the project.* 2. Being or occurring in a disordered or haphazard fashion: W*illy-nilly zoning laws.*

2A6: An enzyme pathway the body uses to metabolize substances.

2B6: An enzyme pathway the body uses to metabolize substances.

2E1: An enzyme pathway the body uses to metabolize substances.

7 RATING: A rating on how you are doing noted in your journal on The Road Back Program. A 7-10 rating is a rating that you are doing well. You are rating how you feel, your energy, appetite, mood and exercise.

REFERENCES

Ambrosone, C. B., Freudenheim J. L., et al. (1999). *"Manganese superoxide dismutase (MnSOD) genetic polymorphisms, dietary antioxidants, and risk of breast cancer."* Cancer Res 59(3): 602-6.

Amores-Sanchez, MI, Medina, MA., *Glutamine, as a precursor of glutathione, and oxidative stress.* Mol Genet Metab 1999;67:100-5.

Aynacioglu, A.S., et al. *Frequency of cytochrome P450 CYP2C9 variants in a Turkish population and functional relevance for phenytoin.* Br J Clin Pharmacol 1999; 48(3):409-415

Bailey, L.B., Gregory, J.F., (1999)."*Polymorphisms of methylenetetrahydrofolate reductase and other enzymes: metabolic significance, risks and impact on folate requirement.*" J Nutr 129(5): 919-22

Bailey, L.B., Gregory, J.F., (1999). "*Folate metabolism and requirements.*" J Nutr 129(4): 779-82

Basile, V.S., Masellis, M., Potkin, S.G., Kennedy, J.L., *Pharmacogenomics in schizophrenia: the quest for individualized therapy.* Hum Mol Genet. 2002 Oct 1;11(20):2517-30

Bertilsson, L., et al (1993) *Molecular basis for rational megaprescribing in ultrarapid hydroxylators of debrisoquine.* Lancet 341:63

Blaisdell, J., Mohrenweiser, H., Jackson, Ferguson, J., Coulter, S., Chanas, S., Chanas, B., Xi, T., Ghanayem, B., Goldstein, J.A. *Identification and functional characterization of new potentially defective alleles of human CYP2C19. Pharmacogenetics.* 2002 Dec;12(9):703-11.

Borgstahl, G. E., H. E. Parge, et al. (1996). "*Human mitochondrial manganese superoxide dismutase polymorphic variant Ile58Thr reduces activity by destabilizing the tetrameric interface.*" Biochemistry 35(14): 4287-97.

Bosron, W.F., Ting-Kai, L., (1986). "*Genetic polymorphism of human liver alcohol and aldehyde dehydrogenases, and their relationship to alcohol metabolism and alcoholism.*" Hepatology 6(3): 502 - 510

Bradford, L.D., *CYP2D6 allele frequency in European Caucasians, Asians, Africans and their descendants.* Pharmacogenomics. 2002 Mar;3 (2):229-43.

Brockmoller, J., et.al. *Pharmacogenetic diagnosis of cytochrome P450 polymorphisms in clinical drug development and in drug treatment.* Pharmacogenetics. 2000:1:125-51.

Bunin, AIa, Filina, A.A., Erchev, V.P., *A glutathione deficiency in open-angle glaucoma and the approaches to its correction.* Vestn Oftalmol 1992;108:13-5 [in Russian].

Cascinu, S., Cordella, L., Del Ferro, E., et al. *Neuroprotective effect of reduced glutathione on cisplatin-based chemotherapy in advanced gastric cancer: a randomized double-blind placebo-controlled trial.* J Clin Oncol 1995;13:26-32.

Ceriello, A., Giugliano, D., Quatraro, A., Lefebvre, P.J., *Anti-oxidants show an anti-hypertensive effect in diabetic and hypertensive subjects.* Clin Sci 1991;81:739-42.

Chang, T.K., et al. *Enhanced cyclophosphamide and ifosfamide activation in primary human hepatocyte cultures: response to cytochrome P-450 inducers and autoinduction by oxazaphosphorines.* Cancer Res 1997; 57(10):1946-54.

Chango, A., Boisson, F., et al. (2000). *"The effect of 677C-->T and 1298A-->C mutations on plasma homocysteine and 5,10-methylenetetrahydrofolate reductase activity in healthy subjects."* Br J Nutr 83(6): 593-6.

Cheng, T., Zhu, Z., et al. (2001). *"Effects of multinutrient supplementation on antioxidant defense systems in healthy human beings."* J Nutr Biochem 12(7): 388-395.

Chida, M., Yokoi, T., Fukui, T., Kinoshita, M., Yokota, J., Kamataki, T., *Detection of three genetic polymorphisms in the 5'-flanking region and intron 1 of human CYP1A2 in the Japanese population.* Jpn J Cancer Res. 1999 Sep;90(9):899-902

Chistyakov, D. A., Savost'anov, et al. (2001). *"Polymorphisms in the Mn-SOD and EC-SOD genes and their relationship to diabetic neuropathy in type 1 diabetes mellitus."* BMC Med Genet 2(1): 4.

Cosma, G., Crofts, F., et al. (1993). *"Relationship between genotype and function of the human CYP1A1 gene."* J Toxicol Environ Health 40(2-3): 309-16.

Cozza, K.L., Armstrong, S.C., Oesterheld, J.R., *Drug Interaction principles for Medical Practice.* American Psychiatric Publishing Inc. (2003)

Crabb, D. W., Edenberg, H. J., et al. (1989). *"Genotypes for aldehyde dehydrogenase deficiency and alcohol sensitivity. The inactive ALDH2(2) allele is dominant."* J Clin Invest 83(1): 314-6.

Crofts, F., Taioli, E., et al. (1994). *"Functional significance of different human CYP1A1 genotypes."* Carcinogenesis 15(12): 2961-3.

Cronin, K. A., Krebs-Smith, S. M., Feuer, E. J., Troiano, R. P., Ballard-Barbash, R., (2001 May). *"Evaluating the impact of population changes in diet, physical activity, and weight status on population risk for colon cancer (United States)".* Cancer Causes Control 12(4):305-16.

Dalhoff K, Ranek L, Mantoni M, Poulsen HE. *Glutathione treatment of hepatocellular carcinoma.* Liver 1992;12:341-3.

Dekou, V., Whincup, P., et al. (2001*). "The effect of the C677T and A1298C polymorphisms in the methylenetetrahydrofolate reductase gene on homocysteine levels in elderly men and women from the British regional heart study."* Atherosclerosis 154(3): 659-66.

De Morais, S.M., Wilkinson, G.R., Blaisdell, J., Nakamura, K., Meyer, U.A., Goldstein, J. *The major genetic defect responsible for the polymorphism of S-mephenytoin metabolism in humans.* J Biol Chem. 1994 Jun 3;269(22):15419-22

De Morais, S.M., Wilkinson, G.R., Blaisdell, J., Meyer, U.A., Nakamura, K., Goldstein, J.A. *Identification of a new genetic defect responsible for the polymorphism of (S)-mephenytoin metabolism in Japanese.* Mol Pharmacol. 1994 Oct;46(4):594-8

Department of Health, London; Stationary Office (2000). *Committee on Medical Aspects of Food and Nutrition Policy. Folic acid and the prevention of disease.*

Donnerstag,,B., Ohlenschläger, Cinatl, J., et al. *Reduced glutathione and S-acetylglutathione as selective apoptosis-inducing agents in cancer therapy.* Cancer Lett 1996;110:63-70.

Eap, C.B., Bender, S., Sirot, E.J., Cucchia, G., Jonzier-Perey, M., Baumann, P., Allorge, D., Broly, F., *Nonresponse to clozapine and ultrarapid CYP1A2 activity: clinical data and analysis of CYP1A2 gene.* Clin Psychopharmacol. 2004 Apr;24(2):214-9

REFERENCES

Aklillu, Eleni, Carrillo, Juan Antonio, Makonnen, Eyasu, Hellman, Karin, Pitarque, Marià, Bertilsson, Ingelman-Sundberg, Leif and Magnus *Genetic Polymorphism of CYP1A2 in Ethiopians Affecting Induction and Expression: Characterization of Novel Haplotypes with Single-Nucleotide Polymorphisms in Intron 1.* 2003 Mol Pharmacol 64:659-669.

Evans, William E. and McLeod, Howard L. *Pharmacogenomics — Drug Disposition, Drug Targets, and Side Effects.* New England Journal of Medicine 2003; 348:538-549.

Faber, M.S., Fuhr, U., *Time response of cytochrome P450 1A2 activity on cessation of heavy smoking.* Clin Pharmacol Ther. 2004 Aug;76(2):178-84.

Favilli, F., Marraccini, P., Iantomasis, T., Vincenzini, M.T., *Effect of orally administered glutathione on glutathione levels in some organs of rats: role of specific transporters.* Br J Nutr 1997;78:293-300.

Fennell, T. R., MacNeela, J. P., et al. (2000). "Hemoglobin adducts from acrylonitrile and ethylene oxide in cigarette smokers: effects of glutathione S-transferase T1-null and M1-null genotypes." Cancer Epidemiol Biomarkers Prev 9(7): 705-12.

Ferguson, R.J., De Morais, Benhamou, S.M., Benhamou, Bouchardy, S., Bouchardy, C., Blaisdell, J., Ibeanu, G., Wilkinson, G.R., Sarich, T.C., Wright, J.M., Dayer, P., Goldstein, J.A. *A new genetic defect in human CYP2C19: mutation of the initiation codon is responsible for poor metabolism of S-mephenytoin.* J Pharmacol Exp Ther. 1998 Jan;284(1):356-61.

Flagg, E.W., Coates, R.J., Jones, D.P., et al. *Dietary glutathione intake and the risk of oral and pharyngeal cancer.* Am J Epidemiol 1994;139:453-65.

Fohr I.O., Prinz-Lnagenohl, R., et al. (2002). "10-Methyleneterahydrofolate reductase genotype determines the plasma homocysteine-lowering effect of supplementation with 5-methyltetrahydrofolate or folic acid in healthy young women." American Journal of Clinical Nutrition 75: 275 - 82

Fontana, R. J., Lown, K. S., et al. (1999). *"Effects of a chargrilled meat diet on expression of CYP3A, CYP1A, and P- glycoprotein levels in healthy volunteers."* Gastroenterology 117(1): 89-98.

Fowke, J.H., Longcope, C., Hebert, J.R., (2000*) "Brassica Vegetable Consumption Shifts Estrogen Metabolism in Healthy Postmenopausal Women."* Cancer Epidemiol Biomarkers Prev 9(8):773-779.

Gao, X., Albena T., Dinkova-Kostova, P., Talalay (2001). *"Powerful and prolonged protection of human retinal pigment epithelial cells, keratinocytes, and mouse leukemia cells against oxidative damage: The indirect antioxidant effects of sulforaphane."* PNAS 98(26): 15221 - 15226.

Garcia-Giralt, E., Perdereau, B., Brixy, F., et al. *Preliminary study of glutathione, L-cysteine and anthocyans (Recancostat Compositum™) in metastatic colorectal carcinoma with malnutrition.* Seventh International Congress on Anti-Cancer Treatment, February 3-6, 1996, Paris, France.

Getahun, S.M., Chung, F.L., (1999). *"Conversion of glucosinolates to isothiocyanates in humans after ingestion of cooked watercress."* Cancer Epidemiology Biomarkers Preview 8(5): 447 - 451.

Giovannucci, E., (1999). *"Nutritional factors in human cancers."* Adv Exp Med Biol 472: 29-42.

Giovannucci, E., Stampfer, M.J., et al. (1998). *"Multivitamin use, folate, and colon cancer in women in the Nurses' Health Study."* Annals of Internal Medicine 129: 517 – 524

Goldstein, J.A., Ishizaki, T., Chiba, K., De Morais, S.M., Bell, D., Krahn, P.M., Evans, D.A. *Frequencies of the defective CYP2C19 alleles responsible for the mephenytoin poor metabolizer phenotype in various Oriental, Caucasian, Saudi Arabian and American black populations.* Pharmacogenetics 1997, 7: 59-64.

Granfors, M.T., Backman, J.T., Neuvonen, M., Neuvonen, P.J., *Ciprofloxacin greatly increases concentrations and hypotensive effect of tizanidine by*

REFERENCES

inhibiting its cytochrome P450 1A2-mediated presystemic metabolism. Clin Pharmacol Ther. 2004 Dec;76(6):598-606

Guttmacher, Alan E. and Collins, Francis S. *Genomic Medicine — A Primer.* New England Journal of Medicine 2002; 347:1512-1520.

Guyonnet, D., Belloir, C., Suschetet, M., Siess, M.H., Le Bon, A.M., (2001) *Antimutagenic activity of organosulfur compounds from Allium is associated with phase II enzyme induction.* Mut Res 496(1-2)135-142

Hagen, T.M., Wierzbicka, G.T., Sillau, A.H., et al. *Fate of dietary glutathione: disposition in the gastrointestinal tract.* Am J Physiol 1990;259(4Pt1):G530-5.

Hamdy, S.I., Hiratsuka, M., Narahara, K., Endo, N., El-Enany, M., Moursi, N., Ahmed, M.S., Mizugaki, M., *Genotyping of four genetic polymorphisms in the CYP1A2 gene in the Egyptian population.* Br J Clin Pharmacol. 2003 Mar;55(3):321-4

Hamman, M.A., Thompson, G.A., Hall, S.D., *Regioselective and stereoselective metabolism of ibuprofen by human cytochrome P450 2C.* Biochem Pharmacol 1997; 54(1):33-41.

Harada, S., Agarwal, D. P., et al. (2001). *"Metabolic and ethnic determinants of alcohol drinking habits and vulnerability to alcohol-related disorder."* Alcohol Clin Exp Res 25(5 Suppl ISBRA): 71S-75S.

Heim, M. and Meyer, U.A., *Genotyping of poor metabolisers of debrisoquine by allele-specific PCR amplification.* Lancet 1990; 336:529-532.

Hibbeln, J.R., Umhau, J.C., Linnoila, M., et al. *A replication study of violent and nonviolent subjects: cerebrospinal fluid metabolites of serotonin and dopamine are predicted by plasma essential fatty acids.* Biol Psychiatry 1998;44:243–9.

Higashi, M.K., Veenstra, D.L., Kondo, L.M., Wittkowsky, A.K., Srinouanprachanh, S.L., Farin, F.M., Rettie, A.E., *Association between CYP2C9 genetic variants and anticoagulation-related outcomes during warfarin therapy.* JAMA. 2002 Apr 3;287(13):1690-8.

Ho, P.C., et al. *Influence of CYP2C9 genotypes on the formation of a hepatotoxic metabolite of valproic acid in human liver microsomes.* Pharmacogenomics J 2003; 3(6):335-42.

Hong, C.C., Tang, B.K., Hammond, G.L., Tritchler, D., Yaffe, M., Boyd, N.F., *Cytochrome P450 1A2 (CYP1A2) activity and risk factors for breast cancer: a cross-sectional study.* Breast Cancer Res. 2004;6(4):R352-65. Epub 2004 May 07

Hunjan, M.K., Evered, D.F. *Absorption of glutathione from the gastrointestinal tract.* Biochim Biophys Acta 1985;815:184-8.

Ibeanu, G.C., Blaisdell, J., Ghanayem, B.I., Beyeler, C., Benhamou, S., Bouchardy, C., Wilkinson, G.R., Dayer, P., Daly, A.K., Goldstein, J.A. *An additional defective allele, CYP2C19*5, contributes to the S-mephenytoin poor metabolizer phenotype in Caucasians.* Pharmacogenetics. 1998 Apr;8(2):129-35.

Ibeanu, G.C., Goldstein, J.A., Meyer, U., Benhamou, S., Bouchardy, C., Dayer ,P., Ghanayem, B.I., Blaisdell, J. *Identification of new human CYP2C19 alleles (CYP2C19*6 and CYP2C19*2B) in a Caucasian poor metabolizer of mephenytoin.* J Pharmacol Exp Ther. 1998 Sep;286(3):1490-5.

Inoue, K., Asao, T., et al. (2000*). "Ethnic-related differences in the frequency distribution of genetic polymorphisms in the CYP1A1 and CYP1B1 genes in Japanese and Caucasian populations."* Xenobiotica 30(3): 285-95.1.

Jacques, P. F., Bostom, A. G., et al. (1996). *"Relation between folate status, a common mutation in methylenetetrahydrofolate reductase, and plasma homocysteine concentrations."* Circulation 93(1): 7-9.

REFERENCES

Joffe, H.V., Johnson, X.R., Longtine, J., Kucher, N. and Goldhaber, S.Z. *Warfarin dosing and Cytochrome P450 2C9 polymorphisms.* Thromb Haemost; 2004 Jun;91(6):1123-8

Johnston, C.S., Meyer, C.G., Srilakshmi, J.C., *Vitamin C elevates red blood cell glutathione in healthy adults.* Am J Clin Nutr 1993;58:103-5.

Jones, D.P., Coates, R.J., Flagg, E.W., et al. *Glutathione in foods listed in the National Cancer Institute's Health Habits and History Food Frequency Questionnaire.* Nutr Cancer 1995;17:57–75.

Julius, M., Lang, C., Gleiberman, L., et al. *Glutathione and morbidity in a community-based sample of elderly.* J Clin Epidemiol 1994;47:1021-6.

Kalow, W. and Grant, D.M., *Pharmacogenetics - The metabolic and molecular bases of inherited disease.* 1995. Scriver CR, et al, eds. New York: McGraw-Hill, Inc., 293-326

Kang, Z. C., Tsai, S. J., et al. (1999). *"Quercetin inhibits benzo[a]pyrene-induced DNA adducts in human Hep G2 cells by altering cytochrome P-450 1A1 gene expression."* Nutr Cancer 35(2): 175-9.

Kirchheiner, J., Brockmoller, J. *Clinical consequences of cytochrome P450 2C9 polymorphisms.* Clin Pharmacol Ther. 2005 Jan;77(1):1-16.

Kirchheiner, J., Brosen, K., Dahl, M.L., et al.: *CYP2D6 and CYP2C19 genotype-based dose recommendations for antidepressants: a first step towards subpopulation-specific dosages.* Acta Psych Scand 2001 Sept;104(3):173-192.

Kirchheiner, J., Tsahuridu, M., Jabrane, W., Roots, I., Brockmoller, J. *The CYP2C9 polymorphism: from enzyme kinetics to clinical dose recommendations.* Personalized Med 2004 1(1) 63-84

Kirchheiner, J., Nickchen, K., Bauer, M., Wong, M.L., Licinio, J., Roots, I., Brockmoller, J. *Pharmacogenetics of antidepressants and antipsychotics:*

the contribution of allelic variations to the phenotype of drug response. Mol Psychiatry. 2004 May;9 (5):442-73.

Kirchheiner, J., et al. *Pharmacogenetics of antidepressants and antipsychotics: the contribution of allelic variations to the phenotype of drug response.* Molecular Psychiatry 2004 9, 442-473

Lam, Y.W.F., Gaedigk, A., Ereshefsy, L., et al: *CYP2D6 inhibition by selective serotonin reuptake inhibitors: analysis of achievable steady-state plasma concentrations and the effect of ultrarapid metabolism at CYP2D6.* Pharmacotherapy 2002;22:1001-1006.

Lampe, J.W., Chen C., et al. (2000). *"Modulation of human glutathione S-transferases by botanically defined vegetable diets."* Cancer Epidemiology Biomarkers Preview 9(8):787-93.

Landi, S., (2000). *"Mammalian class theta GST and differential susceptibility to carcinogens: a review."* Mutat Res 463(3): 247-83.

Lanza, E; Schatzkin, A., Daston, C., Corle, D., Freedman, L., Ballard-Barbash, R., Caan, B., Lance, P., Marshall, J., Iber, F., Shike, M., Weissfeld, J., Slattery, M., Paskett, E., Mateski, D., Albert, P., and the PPT Study Group (2001). *"Implementation of a 4-y, high-fiber, high-fruit-and-vegetable, low-fat dietary intervention: results of dietary changes in the Polyp Prevention Trial 1, 2"* Am J Clin Nutr 74:387-401

Lenzi, A., Picardo, M., Gandini, L., et al. *Glutathione treatment of dyspermia: effect on the lipoperoxidation process.* Hum Reprod 1994;9:2044-50.

Lenzi, A., Culasso, F., Gandini, L., et al. *Placebo-controlled, double-blind, cross-over trial of glutathione therapy in male infertility.* Hum Reprod 1993;8:1657-62.

Lewis, D.F., Lake, B.G., Dickins, M., *Substrates of human cytochromes P450 from families CYP1 and CYP2: analysis of enzyme selectivity and metabolism. Drug* Metabol Drug Interact. 2004;20(3):111-42.

REFERENCES

Lin, H.J., Probst-Hensch, N.M., Louie, A.D., Kau, I.H., Witte, J.S., Ingles, S.A., Frankl, H.D., Lee, E.R., Haile, R.W., (1998 Aug). *"Glutathione transferase null genotype, broccoli, and lower prevalence of colorectal adenomas."* Cancer Epidemiol Biomarkers Prev 7(8):647-52.

Linder, M.W., Prough, R.A., Valdes, R. Jr. Pharmacogenetics: *a laboratory tool for optimizing therapeutic efficiency.* Clin Chem 1997;43:254-66.

Linder, M.W., Valdes, R .Jr. *Pharmacogenetics in the Practice of Laboratory Medicine. Molecular Diagnosis.* 1999;4:365-79.

Linder, M.W., Valdes, R. Jr. *Genetic mechanisms for variability in drug response and toxicity.* J Anal Toxicol 2001;25:405-13.

Linder, M.W., Valdes, R. Jr. *Pharmacogenetics in the practice of laboratory medicine.* Mol Diagn 1999;4:365-79.

Linder, M.W., Valdes, R. Jr. *Fundamentals and applications of pharmacogenetics for the clinical laboratory.* Ann Clin Lab Sci 1999;29:140-9.

London, S. J., Yuan, J. M., et al. (2000). *"Isothiocyanates, glutathione S-transferase M1 and T1 polymorphisms, and lung-cancer risk: a prospective study of men in Shanghai, China."* Lancet 356(9231): 724-9.

Lundqvist, E., Johansson, I., Ingelman-Sundberg, M. *Genetic mechanisms for duplication and multiduplication of the human CYP2D6 gene and methods for detection of duplicated CYP2D6 genes.* Gene 1999 Jan 21;226(2):327-338.

Lutz, W. K., *"Carcinogens in the diet vs overnutrition. Individual dietary habits, malnutrition, and genetic susceptibility modify carcinogenic potency and cancer risk."* Mutation Research (1999) 443: 251-258

Marez, D., Legrand, M., Sabbagh, N., Guidice, J.M., Spire, C., Lafitte, J.J., Meyer, U.A., Broly, F. *Polymorphism of the cytochrome P450 CYP2D6 gene in a European population: characterization of 48 mutations and 53 alleles, their frequencies and evolution.* Pharmacogenetics. 1997 Jun;7(3):193-202.

Michaud, D.S., Spiegelman, D., et al.(1999). *"Fruit and vegetable intake and incidence of bladder cancer in a male prospective cohort."* J Natl Cancer Inst 91(7): 605-13.

Miller, M.C. 3rd, Mohrenweiser, H.W., Bell, D.A. (2001) *"Genetic variability in susceptibility and response to toxicants."* Toxicol Lett 120(1-3):269-80

Miners, J. *CYP2C9 polymorphism: impact on tolbutamide pharmacokinetics and response.* Pharmacogenetics 2002; 12(2):91-2.

Molloy, J., Martin, J.F., Baskerville, P.A., et al. *S-nitrosoglutathione reduces the rate of embolization in humans. Circulation* 1998;98:1372-5.

Nakajima, M., Yokoi, T., Mizutani, M., Kinoshita, M., Funayama, M., Kamataki, T. *Genetic polymorphism in the 5'-flanking region of human CYP1A2 gene: effect on the CYP1A2 inducibility in humans.* J Biochem (Tokyo). 1999 Apr;125(4):803-8

Nemets, B., Stahl, Z., Belmaker,R.H. *Addition of omega-3 fatty acid to maintenance medication treatment for recurrent unipolar depressive disorder.* Am J Psychiatry 2002;159:477–9.

Nijhoff, W.A., Mulder, T.P., et al. (1995*). "Effects of consumption of Brussels sprouts on plasma and urinary glutathione S-transferase class-alpha and -pi in humans."* Carcinogenesis 16(4): 955-7.

Parke, D.V. (1999). *"Antioxidants and disease prevention: mechanisms of action".* Antioxidants in Human Health. CABI Publishing.

Perera, F. P. and Weinstein, I. B. (2000). *"Molecular epidemiology: recent advances and future directions."* Carcinogenesis 21(3): 517-24.

Peyvandi, F., Spreafico, M., Siboni, S.M., Moia, M. and Mannucci, P.M. *CYP2C9 genotypes and dose requirements during the induction phase of oral anticoagulation therapy.* Clinical Pharmacology and Therapeutics 2004; 75(3):198-203

Regier, D.A., Narrow, W.E., Rae, D.S., et al. *The de facto US mental and addictive disorders service system. Epidemiologic Catchment Area prospective 1-year prevalence rates of disorders and services.* Arch Gen Psychiatry 1993;50:85–94.

Rozen, R. (2000). *"Genetic modulation of homocysteinemia."* Semin Thromb Hemost 26(3): 255-61.

Rettie, A.E., et al. *Impaired (S)-warfarin metabolism catalysed by the R144C allelic variant of CYP2C9.* Pharmacogenetics 1994; 4(1):39-42.

Sachse, C., Brockmoller, J., Bauer, S., Roots, I. *Functional significance of a C-->A polymorphism in intron 1 of the cytochrome P450 CYP1A2 gene tested with caffeine.* Br J Clin Pharmacol. 1999 Apr;47(4):445-9

Sandhu, M.S., White, I.R., McPherson, K. (2001). *"Systematic review of the prospective cohort studies on meat consumption and colorectal cancer risk: a meta-analytical approach."* Cancer Epidemiol Biomarkers Prev 10(5): 439-46

Schuppe, H.C., Wieneke, P., Donat, S., Fritsche, E., Kohn, F.M., Abel, J. (2000). *"Xenobiotic metabolism, genetic polymorphisms and male infertility."* Andrologia 32(4-5): 255-62

Scordo, M.G., et al. *Genetic polymorphism of cytochrome P450 2C9 in a Caucasian and a black African population.* Br J Clin Pharmacol 2001; 52(4):447-450.

Sechi, G., Deledda, M.G., Bua, G., et al. *Reduced intravenous glutathione in the treatment of early Parkinson's disease.* Prog Neuropsychopharmacol Biol Psychiatry 1996;20:1159-70.

Sen, C.K. *Nutritional biochemistry of cellular glutathione.* Nutr Biochem 1997;8:660-72.

Sinha, R., Chow, W.H., Kulldorff, M., Denobile, J., Butler, J., Garcia-Closas, M., Weil, R., Hoover, R.N., Rothman, N. (1999). *"Well-done, grilled red meat increases the risk of colorectal adenomas."* Cancer Res 59(17): 4320-4

Smith, T.J., Yang, C.S. (2000). *"Effect of organosulfur compounds from garlic and cruciferous vegetables on drug metabolism enzymes."* Drug Metabol Drug Interact 17(1-4):23-49

Solus, J.F., Arietta, B.J., Harris, J.R., Sexton, D.P., Steward, J.Q., McMunn, C., Ihrie, P., Mehall, J.M., Edwards, T.L., Dawson, E.P. *Genetic variation in eleven phase I drug metabolism genes in an ethnically diverse population.* Pharmacogenomics. 2004 Oct;5(7):895-931.

Spiteri, M. A., Bianco, A., et al. (2000). *"Polymorphisms at the glutathione S-transferase, GSTP1 locus: a novel mechanism for susceptibility and development of atopic airway inflammation."* Allergy 55(Suppl 61): 15-20.

Steen, V.M., et al. *Detection of the poor metabolizer-associated CYP2D6(D) gene deletion by long-PCR technology.* Pharmacogenetics 1995; 5:215-223.

Steinkellner, H., Rabot, S., Freywald, C., Nobis, E., Scharf, G., Chabicovsky, M., Knasmuller, S., Kassie, F. (2001). *"Effects of cruciferous vegetables and their constituents on drug metabolizing enzymes involved in the bioactivation of DNA-reactive dietary carcinogens."* Mutat Res 480-481: 285-97

Stoll, A.L., Severus, W.E., Freeman, M.P., et al. *Omega 3fatty acids in bipolar disorder: a preliminary double-blind, placebo-controlled trial.* Arch Gen Psychiatry 1999;56:407–12.

Strange, R. C., Spiteri, M. A., et al. (2001). *"Glutathione-S-transferase family of enzymes."* Mutat Res 482(1-2): 21-6.

Smyth, J.F., Bowman, A., Perren, T., et al. *Glutathione reduces the toxicity and improves quality of life of women diagnosed with ovarian cancer treated with cisplatin: results of a double-blind, randomised trial.* Ann Oncol 1997;8:569-73.

Takahashi, H., Echizen, H. *Pharmacogenetics of warfarin elimination and its clinical implications.* Clin Pharmacokinet 2001; 40(8):587-603.

Takeshita, T. and Morimoto, K. (2000). *"Accumulation of hemoglobin-associated acetaldehyde with habitual alcohol drinking in the atypical ALDH2 genotype."* Alcohol Clin Exp Res 24(1): 1-7.

Testa, B., Mesolella, M., Testa, D. *Glutathione in the upper respiratory tract.* Ann Otol Rhinol Laryngol 1995;104:117-9.

Trickler, D., Shklar, G., Schwartz, J. *Inhibition of oral carcinogenesis by glutathione.* Nutr Cancer 1993;20:139-44.

Ueland, P. M., Hustad, S., et al. (2001). *"Biological and clinical implications of the MTHFR C677T polymorphism."* Trends Pharmacol Sci 22(4): 195-201.

Vakevainen, S., Tillonen, J., Agarwal, D.P., Srivastava, N., Salaspuro, M. (2000). *"High salivary acetaldehyde after a moderate dose of alcohol in ALDH2-deficient subjects: strong evidence for the local carcinogenic action of acetaldehyde."* Alcohol Clin Exp Res 22(4): 195-201

Van der Weide, J. and Steijns, L.S.W. *Cytochrome P450 enzyme system: genetic polymorphisms and impact on clinical pharmacology.* Ann Clin Biochem 1999; 36:722-729.

Van Iersel, M.L., Verhagen, H., et al. (1999). *"The role of biotransformation in dietary (anti)carcinogenesis."* Mutation Research 443(1-2): 259-70.

Van Landeghem, G. F., Tabatabaie, P., et al. (1999). *"Ethnic variation in the mitochondrial targeting sequence polymorphism of MnSOD."* Hum Hered 49(4): 190-3.

Vendemiale, G., Altomare, E., Trizio, T., et al. *Effects of oral S-adenosyl-L-methionine on hepatic glutathione in patients with liver disease. Scand J Gastroenterol* 1989;24:407-15.

Verhoeff, B. J., Trip, M. D., et al. (1998). *"The effect of a common methylenetetrahydrofolate reductase mutation on levels of homocysteine, folate, vitamin B12 and on the risk of premature atherosclerosis."* Atherosclerosis 141(1): 161-6.

Wang, S.T., Chen, H.W., Sheen, L.Y., Lii, C.K. *Methionine and cysteine affect glutathione level, glutathione-related enzyme activities and the expression of glutathione S-transferase isozymes in rat hepatocytes. J Nutr* 1997;127:2135-41.

Wang, X., Zuckerman, B., et al. (2002) *"Maternal cigarette smoking, metabolic gene polymorphism, and infant birth weight."* Journal of the American Medical Association 287(2): 195 - 202

Weinshilboum, Richard. *Inheritance and Drug Response* New England Journal of Medicine 2003; 348:529-537

White, A.C., Thannickal, V.J., Fanburg, B.L. *Glutathione deficiency in human disease. J Nutr Biochem* 1994;5:218–26.

Willett, W.C. (1995). *"Diet, nutrition, and avoidable cancer"*. Environ Health Perspect 103(Suppl 8): 165-170

Williams, J.A., Martin, F.L., Muir, G.H., Hewer, A., Grover, P.L., Phillips, D.H. (2000). *"Metabolic activation of carcinogens and expression of various cytochromes P450 in human prostate tissue."* Carcinogenesis 21(9): 1683-9.

Witschi, A., Reddy, S., Stofer, B., Lauterburg, B.H. *The systemic availability of oral glutathione. Eur J Clin Pharmacol* 1992;43:667-9.

Wolf ,C.R. and Smith, G. *Pharmacogenetics.* Br Med Bull 1999; 55(2):366-386.

Xiao, Z.S., Goldstein, J.A., Xie, H.G., Blaisdell, J., Wang, W., Jiang, C.H., Yan, F.X., He, N., Huang, S.L., Xu, Z.H., Zhou, H.H. *Differences in the incidence of the CYP2C19 polymorphism affecting the S-mephenytoin phenotype in Chinese Han and Bai populations and identification of a new rare CYP2C19 mutant allele.* J Pharmacol Exp Ther. 1997 Apr;281(1):604-9.

Yamauchi, M., Takeda, K., Sakamoto, K., Searashi, Y., Uetake, S., Kenichi, H., Toda, G. (2001). *"Association of polymorphism in the alcohol dehydrogenase 2 gene with alcohol-induced testicular atrophy."* Alcohol Clin Exp Res 25(Suppl 6): 16-8

Yokoyama, A., Muramatsu, T., Ohmori, T., Yokoyama, T., Okuyama, K., Takahashi, H., Hasegawa, Y., Higuchi, S., Maruyama, K., Shirakura, K., Ishii, H. (1998). *"Alcohol-related cancers and aldehyde dehydrogenase-2 in Japanese alcoholics."* Carcinogenesis 19(8):1383-7

Zackrisson, A.L., Lindblom, B. *Identification of CYP2D6 alleles by single nucleotide polymorphism analysis using pyrosequencing.* Eur J Clin Pharmacol. 2003 Oct;59 (7):521-6.

Zhao, B., Seow, A, Lee, E.J., Poh, W.T., The, M., Eng, P., Wang, Y.T., Tan, W.C., Yu, M.C., Lee, H.P. (2001*). "Dietary isothiocyanates, glutathione S-transferase -M1, -T1 polymorphisms and lung cancer risk among Chinese women in Singapore."* Cancer Epidemiol Biomarkers Prev 10(10): 1063-7

Zusterzeel, P.L., Nelen, W.L., Roelofs, H.M., Peters, W.H., Blom, H.J., Steegers, E.A. (2000). *"Polymorphisms in biotransformation enzymes and the risk for recurrent early pregnancy loss."* Mol Hum Reprod 6(5): 474-8

FLOW CHART

PRE-TAPER FLOW CHART
IF YOU HAVE DAYTIME ANXIETY,
AGITATION OR INSOMNIA WHILE
TAKING CYMBALTA

STEP 1

GOAL: Improved sleep
Vast reduction or elimination of anxiety
A lessening or elimination of other medication-induced side effects

Supplements you will take:
Essential Protein Formula, Body Calm, Body Calm Supreme,
Beta 1,3-D Glucan

DAY ONE:
Action: Rate your daytime anxiety, panic attacks, insomnia and other side effects in your Daily Journal. Rate   number 1 being the worst and 10 being no side effect or symptom remaining.
Take: Essential Protein Formula: 1 tsp mixed in the liquid of your choice
Body Calm Supreme: 1 capsule
Time: At bedtime

continued➡

STEP 1
(continued)

DAY 2, 3 & 4
Action: Rate your daytime anxiety, panic attacks, insomnia and other side effects in your Daily Journal from 1-10. Number 1 being the worst and 10 being no side effect or symptom remaining.
Rate the previous night sleep first thing the next morning
Rate daytime anxiety just before bedtime of that day.
Take: Essential Protein: 1 tsp mixed in a liquid of your choice
Body Calm Supreme: 1 capsule
Time: First thing in the morning when you awaken
Take: Beta 1, 3-D Glucan: 1 capsule 100mg
Time: Any time in the morning. Make sure to only use as much liquid as needed to wash the capsule down and do not have any other liquid or food for ½ hour after taking the supplements. Ideally you would not have food 1/2 hour before taking the Beta 1, 3-D Glucan.

The rest of the day and up until bedtime you will be alternating the Body Calm and the Body Calm Supreme every 4 hours
Example:
7am: or when you awaken 1 Body Calm Supreme and 1 tsp Essential Protein
11am: 1 Body Calm capsule and 1 tsp of Essential Protein
3pm: 1 Body Calm Supreme capsule and 1 tsp Essential Protein
7pm: 1 Body Calm capsule and 1 tsp of Essential Protein
11pm: or at bedtime 1 Body Calm Supreme capsule and 1 tsp Essential Protein

DAY 5:
Action: The morning of day 5: Rate your sleep from the night before and have a look at your Daily Journal regarding daytime anxiety. If you now rate your daytime anxiety at a 7 or higher and your sleep is at a 7 or higher, proceed to **Step 2.**

If you do not rate yourself at a 7 or higher for daytime anxiety and sleep locate the scenario that fits your circumstance to right.

STEP 2

Continue taking all supplements as established during Step1
GOAL: Improvement of mood
A lessening or elimination of other medication induced side effects
SUPPLEMENT YOU WILL INTRODUCE:
Ultimate Omega 3

DAY 1:
ACTION: Use your Daily Journal and rate your mood and any additional symptoms from 1-10
TAKE: 4 Ultimate Omega 3 soft gels
TIME: 2 First thing in the morning and 2 around noon, but before 4pm

DAY 2, 3 &4:
ACTION: Use your Daily Journal and rate your mood and any additional symptoms from 1-10
TAKE: 6 Ultimate Omega 3 soft gels
TIME: 3 First thing in the morning when you awaken and 3 around noon, but before 4pm

You are finished with Step 2 now go to Step 3

STEP 3

Continue taking all supplements as established during Steps 1 and 2
GOAL: Overall brightness of feelings and mood
Nice and smooth energy level
A lessening or elimination of other medication induced side effects
SUPPLEMENT YOU WILL INTRODUCE:
RenewPro

DAY 1:
ACTION: Use your Daily Journal and rate your mood, anxiety, sleep and any additional symptoms you may be experiencing from 1-10. Rate with number 1 being the worst and number 10 being no side effect or symptom remaining
TAKE: ½ scoop of RenewPro
TIME: First thing in the morning

DAY2,3 & 4:
ACTION: Use your Daily Journal and rate your anxiety, sleep and any additional symptoms you may be experiencing from 1-10.
TAKE: ½ scoop of RenewPro
TIME: First thing in the morning and around noon

You are finished with Step 3 now go to Step 4

STEP 4
DAY 1:

ACTION: Begin taking 400 i.u. of vitamin E first thing in the morning with the rest of your morning supplements. Begin taking 1 capsule of Nature's Vitamin C any time around midday. **If you are taking ADHD medication do not take any vitamin C and watch your fruit intake**

Keep taking all supplements exactly as you
have established during the pre-taper.

You are completely finished with the pre-taper when:

22 days have passed after you started Step 1
And
You rated yourself at a 7 or higher for anxiety and sleep

You do need to wait the 22 days from the date you started Step 1, even if you are at a 7 rating or higher for anxiety and insomnia.

Continue taking all supplements exactly as you are now during the tapering portion of the medication.

If you have tried to quit these medications in the past you may be a little apprehensive about reducing the medication again. You can remain at this stage of the process for as long as you like. You do not have to rush.

When you are ready, follow the procedures detailed in the chapter, "How to Taper Off Antidepressants, Antipsychotics and ADHD Medication (Slow and Gradual)" or the next chapter "How to Taper Off Antidepressants, Antipsychotics and ADHD Medication (Fast and Gradual)."

PROBLEMS YOU MAY RUN INTO AND HOW TO HANDLE

IF YOU ARE HAVING DIFFICULTY GOING TO SLEEP:

- Try taking all the supplements ½ hour before bedtime for 3 nights. If still no change, try taking the supplements 1 hour before bedtime for 3 nights. If you begin to feel tired before your normal bedtime go to bed a little earlier than usual. This may be your window of opportunity for going to sleep with ease and we do not want to miss the chance.

IF YOU ARE WAKING UP IN THE MIDDLE OF THE NIGHT AND ARE HAVING DIFICULTY GOING BACK TO SLEEP:

- If you are waking up in the middle of the night and are able to go back to sleep with little effort that is very normal. If you have difficulty going back to sleep take 1 Body Calm Supreme in the night when you awaken.

IF YOU BEGIN TO SLEEP WELL WITH A 7 OR HIGHER RATING, BUT WAKE UP TIRED:

- Reduce the last supplement that was increased slightly. You can open up any of the capsules and remove ½ of the supplement powder.

OTHER OPTIONS

There are other options available with using the Body Calm, Body Calm Liquid and the Body Calm Supreme. The next section provides further ways an individual may use, change or alter these products for anxiety and or insomnia.

- ***Body Calm*** — You can add 1 Body Calm capsule with each Body Calm Supreme if needed. You can take as many as 3 Body Calm capsules at bedtime for sleep.

- ***Body Calm Liquid*** — For some, but very few, the Body Calm liquid was the answer for the daytime anxiety and or insomnia. Making the switch from capsule to liquid can be magic.

- ***Body Calm Supreme*** — As described in the chapter "General Pre-Tapering and Tapering Instructions" reaching a "steady state" can be different for each person. If you are feeling some relief from anxiety, but it is only temporary, you may need to change the frequency or amount of Body Calm Supreme. You can take the Body Calm Supreme every 2 hours during the day to achieve this. For some people this made astounding results.

- ***Pro Biotic Supreme***—If you have not added the Probiotic Supreme to your daily supplements, you might have Candida yeast overgrowth. You can take 2 capsules of the Probiotic Supreme any time during the day with food. If you use birth control pills or have taken an antibiotic in the past, we do urge you to use the Probiotic Supreme for the 60-days. Adding the Probiotic Supreme for 60-days may just be the assistance your body needs.

If you have felt any improvement during these procedures, you have something to work with. If the anxiety has at least moved from a rating of 3 to 5 and the anxiety is holding at that level using these supplements will be the answer for your success. You just need to adjust them further, allow a little additional time or adjust the time of day you are taking them. Adjust supplements one-by-one every third day. Keep good notes in your journal. The answers will either be the quantity taken of a supplement or it will be how often the supplement is taken.

Experiment with this as needed and keep your Daily Journal. Give this some time to work. If you have had some improvement, such as from a 3 to a 5 rating and it is holding steady, but will not move beyond a 5 rating move on to Step 2 and keep rating the daytime anxiety each evening. It may very well improve to a 7 rating later in the pre-taper.

ONE OF THESE 9 THINGS IS HAPPENING

IF YOU COMPLETE ALL STAGES FOR ANXIETY AND SLEEP AND YOU STILL RATE ANXIETY AND SLEEP BELOW A 7 ON A 1-10 SCALE, ONE OF THESE NINE THINGS ARE OUT:

- You are one of the few who need to continue taking the supplements for additional time before they will work for you. This does happen but is rare.

- You need to reevaluate how you are rating yourself. Are you being a little too rough on yourself? How are you judging yourself?

- Reread the section in the chapter, "General Pre-Tapering and Tapering Instructions."

- Keep in mind, if you had anxiety throughout the day and the anxiety was extreme and the anxiety is now only in the morning when you wake up and then disappears for the rest of the day, you have had a major positive change.

- Review all the sleep scenarios in the chapter, "General Pre-Tapering and Tapering Instructions." Before starting Step 1 of the Pre-Taper, if you use to wake up in the middle of the night and had a difficult time going back to sleep, but now you wake up in the middle of the night and instantly go back to sleep, this is a major positive change.

- You are taking other supplements and the real reason you will not respond to Stage 1 is the other supplements. This is when you need to reevaluate calcium, if you are taking it, B vitamins, and all

- other supplements. The other supplements, herbs or other concoctions may have been causing the increased anxiety or insomnia for some time.

- These other supplements might be excellent but not when you are taking medication from this group.

- See your doctor. Ask your doctor if you can quit taking the other supplements that are not part of The Road Back Program. If this is fine with your doctor, discontinue the other supplements. Continue taking the supplements used during Step 1 of the Pre-Taper. Give yourself 3 days and see how you are doing.

- You are changing something.

- You are not taking the supplements as outlined.

- Maybe you are changing the time of day when you take your medication.

- Look at the weekends. Are you sleeping in a few hours later and not taking the morning medication at the same time? Are you staying up later in the evening and not taking the medication at the same time?

- Have you changed your daily routine?

- You started The Road Back Program after you have already made one or several attempts to come off your medication and you were having withdrawal side effects before starting the program.

- You should give Step 1 additional time. Many people respond quickly to this step, even if they fit into this category, but some require from 14 to 30 days to fully complete Step 1 when they fall in this group.

- I suggest that you give it some time, at least the 30 days.

- The Road Back Program is not for you. I wish I could say this program works for everyone, but it does not. From 8 years experience, I know the percentage is very low that this program will not work for, but there is that percentage, nonetheless.

At least you have not caused additional harm by your attempt.

FLOW CHART

PRE-TAPER IF YOU HAVE FATIGUE AND DO NOT HAVE ANXIETY OR INSOMNIA

STEP 1

SUPPLEMENT YOU WILL INTRODUCE:
Power Barley
You will be increasing the Power Barley Formula slowly over a number of days. At any time during the pre-taper when you feel an increased energy a new brightness about yourself, an overall good feeling, **DO NOT INCREASE THE POWER BARLEY FORMULA FURTHER**.

DAY 1:
ACTION: In your Daily Journal rate your fatigue, mood, anxiety, sleep and any additional symptoms you may be experiencing from 1-10. Rate number 1 being the worst and 10 being no side effect or symptom remaining.
TAKE: Power Barley Formula: ½ teaspoon
TIME: First thing in the morning

continued➡

STEP 1
(continued)

DAY 2,3 & 4:
ACTION: In your Daily Journal rate your fatigue, anxiety, sleep and all side effects.
TAKE: Power Barley Formula: ½ teaspoon
TIME: First thing in the morning around noon and once again before 4pm

DAY 5,6 &7:
ACTION: Rate your fatigue, anxiety, sleep and all side effects in your Daily Journal from 1-10
TAKE: Power Barley Formula: 1 teaspoon
TIME: First thing in the morning, around noon and once again before 4 pm

DAY 8,9&10:
ACTION: Rate your fatigue, anxiety, sleep and all side effects in your Daily Journal
TAKE: Power Barley Formula: 2 teaspoons
TIME: First thing in the morning, around noon and once again before 4 pm

DAY 11,12&13:
ACTION: Rate your fatigue, anxiety, sleep and all side effects in your Daily Journal.
TAKE: Power Barley Formula: 1 tablespoon
TIME: First thing in the morning, around noon and once again before 4 pm

YOU ARE NOW READY TO MOVE TO STEP 2 →

STEP 2

Continue taking all supplements as established during Step 1

GOAL: Improvement of mood
A lessening or elimination of other medication induced side effects

SUPPLEMENT YOU WILL INTRODUCE:
Ultimate Omega 3

DAY 1:
ACTION: Rate your mood and other side effects in your Daily Journal
TAKE: 2 Ultimate Omega 3 softgels
TIME: 2 first thing in the morning and 2 around noon but before 4pm

DAY 2,3 & 4:
ACTION: Rate your mood and other side effects in your Daily Journal.
TAKE: 4 Ultimate Omega 3 softgels
TIME: 4 first thing in the morning when you wake up and 4 around noon, but before 4pm

YOU ARE NOW READY TO MOVE TO STEP 3 →

STEP 3

Continue taking all supplements as established during Step 1 and 2

GOAL: Improved sleep
A vast reduction or elimination of anxiety
A lessening or elimination of other medication-induced side effects

SUPPLEMENTS YOU WILL INTRODUCE:
Essential Protein Formula
Body Calm
Body Calm Supreme

DAY 1:
ACTION: Rate your daytime mood, anxiety, panic attacks, insomnia, fatigue and other side effects in your Daily Journal. Rate with number 1 being the worst and number 10 being no side effect at all
TAKE: Essential Protein Formula: 1 tsp mixed in a liquid of your choice
TIME: At bedtime

DAY 2, 3 & 4:
ACTION: Rate your daytime mood anxiety, panic attacks, insomnia, fatigue and other side effects in your Daily Journal. Rate with number 1 being the worst and 10 being no side effect or symptom. Rate the previous night's sleep first thing the next morning and daytime anxiety before bedtime of that day.
TAKE: Essential Protein Formula: 1 tsp mixed in a liquid of your choice
Body Calm Supreme: 1 capsule
TIME: First thing in the morning when you awake

The rest of the day and up until bedtime you will be alternating the Body Calm Supreme and the Body Calm every 4 hours.

EXAMPLE:

7am: or when you awaken 1 Body Calm Supreme and 1 tsp Essential Protein Formula

11am: 1 Body Calm and 1 tsp Essential Protein Formula

3pm: 1 Body Calm Supreme and 1 tsp Essential **Protein Formula**

7pm: 1Body Calm and 1 tsp Essential Protein Formula

11pm: or bedtime 1 Body Calm Supreme 1 tsp Essential Protein Formula

STEP 4

DAY 1

Begin taking 400 i.u. of vitamin E first thing in the morning with the rest of morning supplements

Begin taking 1capsule Nature's Vitamin C around noon. **DO NOT TAKE VITAMIN C IF TAKING ADHD MEDICATION.**

IF YOU ARE STILL FEELING ANY DEPRESSION:

You can take up to 3 softgels of CLA daily. Take 1 in the morning, one near noon and the 3rd before 4pm.

If you have not added Probiotic Supreme to your daily supplements you might have Candida yeast overgrowth. Adding Probiotic Supreme for 60-days may be the assistance your body needs.

You can add up to 2 full scoops of RenewPro each day to your routine.

Keep taking all supplements exactly as you have established during the pre-taper.

You are completely finished with the pre-taper when:
22-days have passed after your started Step 1
And
You rate yourself at a 7 or higher for anxiety and sleep

Continue taking all supplements exactly as you are now during the tapering portion of the program.

If you have tried to quit these medications in the past you may be a little apprehensive about reducing the medication again. You can remain at this stage of the process for as long as you like. You do not have to rush.

You now need to make a decision on which taper to follow. You can taper off the medication twice as fast with this program if desired The slower method has been kept in the book for those of you wishing to really take your time with the taper portion.

The two chapters are the following:

"How to Taper Off Antidepressants, Antipsychotics and ADHD Medication (Slow and Gradual)" or "How to Taper Off Antidepressants, Antipsychotics and ADHD Medication (Fast and Gradual Taper)".

FLOW CHART

PRE-TAPER BENZODIAZEPINES, ANTI-ANXIETY, ANTICONVULSANT AND SLEEP MEDICATION

STEP 1

GOALS: Improved sleep
Vast reduction or elimination of anxiety
Lessening or elimination of other medication-induced side effects

SUPPLEMENTS YOU WILL TAKE:
Essential Protein Formula
Body Calm
Body Calm Supreme
Beta 1, 3-D Glucan (100mg each)

DAY 1:
ACTION: On your Daily Journal rate your daytime anxiety, insomnia and other side effects.
Rate with number 1 being the worst and number 10 being no side effect or symptom remaining.
TAKE: Essential Protein Formula 1 tsp mixed in a liquid of your choice
1 Body Calm Supreme capsule
TIME: At bedtime

continued➙

STEP 1
(continued)

DAY 2, 3&4:
ACTION: On your Daily Journal rate your daytime anxiety, insomnia, panic attacks and other side effects from 1-10.
Rate the previous night sleep first thing in the morning when you awaken
Rate daytime anxiety just before bedtime of that day
TAKE: Essential Protein Formula 1 tsp mixed in liquid of your choice
Body Calm Supreme 1 capsule
TIME: First thing in the morning when you awaken
TAKE: Beta 1, 3-D Glucan 2 capsules 100mg each
TIME: Any time in the morning. Make sure you only use enough liquid to wash down the capsules and do not have any liquid or food for ½ hour later. Ideally you would not have food ½ hour before taking Beta 1, 3-D Glucan.
11pm or bedtime 1 Body Calm Supreme, 1 tsp Essential Protein

The rest of the day and up until bedtime you will be alternating the Body Calm Supreme and the Body Calm every 4 hours.

EXAMPLE:
> 7am: or when you awaken 1 Body Calm Supreme, 1 tsp Essential Protein
> 11am: 1 Body Calm, 1 tsp Essential Protein
> 3pm: 1 Body Calm Supreme, 1 tsp Essential Protein
> 7pm: 1 Body Calm, 1 tsp Essential Protein

DAY 5:
ACTION: Rate your sleep from the night before and have a look at your Daily Journal regarding daytime anxiety. **IF YOU NOW RATE YOUR DAYTIME ANXIETY AND SLEEP AT A 7 OR HIGHER RATING GO TO STEP 2.**

STEP 2
DAYTIME ANXIETY
7 OR HIGHER
SLEEP 7 OR HIGHER
(page 272)

FLOW CHARTS

**DAYTIME ANXIETY BELOW A 7 RATING
AND SLEEP AT A 7 OR HIGHER:**

Replace Body Calm with Body Calm Supreme during the day and continue Essential protein every 4 hours. Rate your anxiety and sleep if at a 7 or higher for 3 consecutive days move to Step 2. If not continue to the next step below.

**IF YOU ARE NOT AT A 7 OR HIGHER AFTER 8 FULL
DAYS FOLLOWING THE PREVIOUS STEP:**

Continue the supplements from the previous step. Increase Essential Protein to 4 tsp every 4 hours. Increase Beta 1 3-D Glucan to 2 capsules in the am, 2 around noon and 2 in the late afternoon. Do not consume liquid or food ½ hour after taking Beta 1 3-D Glucan. Ideally no food ½ hour before. If you rate yourself at a 7 or higher for 3 consecutive days go to Step 2

**DAYTIME ANXIETY ABOVE A 7 RATING
AND SLEEP BELOW A 7 RATING:**

Continue all supplements from Step 1 Increase Body Calm Supreme to 2 capsules at bedtime. 2 additional Beta 1 3-D Glucan after 4pm but before 8pm. If you rate yourself at a 7 or higher for 3 consecutive days move to Step 2. If not continue with the next step below.

**IF YOU ARE STILL AT A DAYTIME ANXIETY ABOVE 7
AND SLEEP BELOW 7:**

Include 1 Body Calm capsule with 2 Body Calm Supreme and 1 tsp of Essential Protein every 4 hours. Continue with the additional Beta 1 3-D Glucan.

DAYTIME ANXIETY BELOW 7 AND SLEEP BELOW A 7 RATING:

Continue all supplements from Step 1.
Replace Body Calm with Body Calm Supreme during the day.
2 additional Beta 1 3-D Glucan after 4pm but before 8pm. If you rate yourself at a 7 or higher for 3 consecutive days move to Step 2. If not continue with the next step.

HOW TO GET OFF CYMBALTA SAFELY

IF NO CHANGE OR YOU ARE STILL NOT UP TO A 7 RATING FOR ANXIETY DO THE FOLLOWING:

Decrease the Essential Protein back down to 1 tsp every 4 hours. Keep taking the Beta 1 3-D Glucan 3 times per day. Increase Body Calm Supreme to 1 capsule every 3 hours. Continue this for 3 full days. Make sure to rate yourself in your Daily Journal. If you have 3 consecutive days of a 7 or higher rating for daytime anxiety move to Step 2. If not continue below.

IF NO CHANGE IN 3 NIGHTS:

Increase Body Calm capsules to 2 at bedtime with 2 Body Calm Supreme and 1 tsp of Essential Protein. Continue with the Beta 1 3-D Glucan. If sleep improves to a 7 or higher for 3 consecutive nights move to Step 2. If not continue with the next step below.

IF NO CHANGE OR SLEEP STILL BELOW A 7 RATING:

Go to "PROBLEMS YOU MAY RUN INTO AND HOW TO HANDLE" If you now have a 7 rating for sleep for 3 consecutive days go to Step 2. If not go to "ONE OF THESE 9 THINGS IS HAPPENING". Handle anything that needed to be handled and move to Step 2.

DAYTIME ANXIETY AND SLEEP STILL BELOW A 7 RATING:

Increase Body Calm Supreme to 1 capsule every 2 hours during the day. 1 tsp Essential protein with Body Calm Supreme Probiotic Supreme as directed on the bottle each day. Nature's Vitamin C, 1 in the am, 1 at noon and 1 before 4pm. CLA, 1 in the am, 1 at 4pm Ultimate Omega 3, 1 in the am, 1 at noon and 1 at 4pm. Vitamin E, 1 in the am Make sure you keep your Daily Journal filled out daily with your 1-10 rating. If you do not rate yourself at a 7 or higher after 7 full days using this approach move to Step 3. Step 3 supplements may be what will get you over the top.

IF YOU COMPLETE ALL STAGES FOR ANXIETY AND SLEEP AND YOU STILL RATE ANXIETY AND SLEEP BELOW A 7 RATING:

See "OTHER OPTIONS", and "PROBLEMS YOU MAY RUN INTO AND HOW TO HANDLE" and "ONE OF THESE 9THINGS IS HAPPENING".

FLOW CHARTS

IF DAYTIME ANXIETY IS STILL NOT RATED AT A 7 OR HIGHER:

Go to "OTHER OPTIONS" If "Other Options" handled your situation and you are now at a 7 or higher go to Step 2

IF DAYTIME ANXIETY IS STILL NOT RATED AT A 7 OR HIGHER:

Go to "PROBLEMS YOU MAY RUN INTO AND HOW TO HANDLE" If this handled your daytime anxiety move to Step 2. If not go to "ONE OF THESE 9 THINGS IS HAPPENING". Handle anything that needs to be handled and move to Step 2.

STEP 2

Continue taking all supplements as established in Step 1

GOALS: Improvement of mood
A lessening or elimination of other medication induced side effects

SUPPLEMENT YOU WILL INTRODUCE:
Ultimate Omega 3

DAY 1:
ACTION: Keep rating anxiety and sleep and rate your mood and other side effects in your Daily Journal. Rate with number 1 being the worst and number 10 being no side effect or symptom remaining.
TAKE: 1 Ultimate Omega 3 softgel
TIME: First thing in the morning and around noon but before 4pm

DAY 2, 3 & 4:
ACTION: Rate your mood, anxiety, sleep and any other side effects you may be experiencing in your Daily Journal from 1-10.
TAKE: 2 Ultimate Omega 3 softgels
TIME: First thing in the morning when you awaken and around noon but before 4pm

NOW YOU CAN MOVE TO STEP 3 →

STEP 3

Continue taking all supplements as established during steps 1 and 2

GOALS: Overall brightness of feelings and mood
Nice and smooth energy level
A lessening or elimination of other medication-induced side effects

SUPPLEMENT YOU WILL INTRODUCE:
RenewPro

DAY 1:
ACTION: In your Daily Journal rate anxiety, sleep, mood and any additional symptoms you may be experiencing.
TAKE: ½ scoop of RenewPro
TIME: First thing in the morning

DAY 2, 3 & 4:
ACTION: In your Daily Journal rate your anxiety, sleep, mood and any additional symptoms you may be experiencing from 1-10. Rate with number 1 being the worst and 10 being no side effect or symptom remaining.
TAKE: ½ scoop of RenewPro
TIME: First thing in the morning, around noon and one more before 4pm

NOW YOU ARE READY TO MOVE TO STEP 4 →

STEP 4

DAY 1:

TAKE: 400 i.u. Vitamin E
TIME: First thing in the morning with the rest of the morning supplements

Keep taking all supplements exactly as you have established during the pre-taper while you taper off the medication and continue for 45 days after the last dosage of medication

You are completely finished with the pre-taper when:
You rate yourself at a 7 or higher for anxiety and sleep.

It is now time to decide which taper program to follow. You can taper off the medication twice as fast with this program if desired. The slower method has been kept in the book for those of you wishing to really take your time with the taper portion.
The two chapters are the following:

How to Taper Off Benzodiazepines, Anti-anxiety, Anticonvulsant and Sleep Medication
(The Slow and Gradual Taper)

How to Taper Off Benzodiazepines, Anti-anxiety, Anticonvulsant and Sleep Medication
(The Fast and Gradual Taper)

PROBLEMS YOU MAY RUN INTO AND HOW TO HANDLE

IF YOU ARE HAVING DIFFICULTY GOING TO SLEEP:

Try taking all the supplements ½ hour before bedtime for 3 nights. If still no change, try taking the supplements 1 hour before bedtime for 3 nights. If you begin to feel tired before your normal bedtime go to bed a little earlier than usual. This may be your window of opportunity for going to sleep with ease and we do not want to miss the chance.

IF YOU ARE WAKING UP IN THE MIDDLE OF THE NIGHT AND ARE HAVING DIFICULTY GOING BACK TO SLEEP:

If you are waking up in the middle of the night and are able to go back to sleep with little effort that is very normal. If you have difficulty going back to sleep take 1 Body Calm Supreme in the night when you awaken.

IF YOU BEGIN TO SLEEP WELL WITH A 7 OR HIGHER RATING, BUT WAKE UP TIRED:

Reduce the last supplement that was increased slightly. You can open up any of the capsules and remove ½ of the supplement powder.

ONE OF THESE 9 THINGS IS HAPPENING

IF YOU COMPLETE ALL STAGES FOR ANXIETY AND SLEEP AND YOU STILL RATE ANXIETY AND SLEEP BELOW A 7 ON A 1-10 SCALE, ONE OF THESE 9 THINGS IS HAPPENING:

1. You are one of the few who need to continue taking the supplements for additional time before they work for you. This does happen but is rare.

2. You need to reevaluate how you are rating yourself. Are you being a little too rough on yourself and how are you judging yourself?

   Reread the section in the chapter, "General Pre-Tapering and Tapering Instructions".

   Keep in mind, if you had anxiety throughout the day and the anxiety was extreme and the anxiety now occurs only in the morning when you wake up and then disappears for the rest of the day, you have had a major positive change.

3. You are taking other supplements and the real reason you will not respond to Stage 1 is the other supplements. This is where you need to reevaluate calcium, if you are taking it, B vitamins, and all other supplements. The other supplements, herbs or concoctions may have been causing the increased anxiety or insomnia for some time.

   These other supplements might be excellent, but not when you are taking medication from this group.

   Meet with your doctor. Ask him or her if you can quit taking the other supplements that are not part of The Road Back Program. If this is ok with your doctor, discontinue the other supplements. Continue taking the supplements used during Step 1 of the Pre-Taper. Give yourself 3 days and see how you are doing.

4. You are changing something. **Have you changed anything in your daily routine?**

5. You are not taking the supplements as outlined.

6. Maybe you are changing the time of day when you take your medication.

7. Look at the weekends. Are you sleeping in a few hours later and not taking the morning medication at the same time? Are you stay-

ing up later in the evening and not taking the medication at the same time?

8. You have started The Road Back Program after you have already made one or several attempts to come off you medication and you were having withdrawal before starting the program.

   You should give Step 1 additional time. Many people respond quickly to this step even if they fit into this category, but some require from 14 to 30 days to fully complete Step 1 when they fall into this group. **I suggest you give it some time, at least 30 days.**

9. The Road Back Program is not for you. I wish I could say this program works for everyone, but it does not. From 8 years experience, I know the percentage of people is very low that this program will not work for, but there is that percentage, nonetheless.

At least you have not caused additional harm by your attempt.

OTHER OPTIONS

There are other options available with using the Body Calm, Body Calm Liquid and the Body Calm Supreme. The next section provides further ways an individual may use, change or alter these products for anxiety and/or insomnia relief.

- *Body Calm capsules* - You can add 1 Body Calm capsule with each Body Calm Supreme if needed. You may take as many 3 Body Calm capsules at bedtime for sleep. You may take 1 Body Calm Supreme along with the Body Calm at bedtime if needed.

- *Body Calm liquid* - For some, but very few, the Body Calm liquid is the answer for the daytime anxiety and/or insomnia. Making the switch from capsule to liquid can be magic.

- ***Body Calm Supreme*** – As described in the chapter "General Pre-Tapering and Tapering Instructions," reaching a "steady state" can be different for each person. If you are feeling some relief from anxiety, but it is only temporary you may need to change the frequency or amount of Body Calm Supreme. You can take the Body Calm Supreme every 2 hours during the day to achieve this. For some people, this gives astounding results.

- ***Nature's Vitamin C—*** As mentioned earlier in this chapter you can take the Nature's Vitamin C and Probiotic Supreme. If the adrenals need help the Nature's Vitamin C would be the supplement to introduce. The adrenals require ample supply of vitamin C to work properly.

- ***Pro Biotic Supreme***—If you have not added the Probiotic Supreme to your daily supplements, you might have Candida yeast overgrowth. You can take 2 capsules of the Probiotic Supreme any time during the day with food. If you use birth control pills or have taken an antibiotic in the past, we do urge you to use the Probiotic Supreme for the 60-days. Adding the Probiotic Supreme for 60-days may just be the assistance your body needs. Most medications will create a yeast overgrowth and the Probiotic Supreme is designed t handle tat quickly. Side effects from yeast overgrowth can include anxiety, depression and insomnia.

- ***CLA—*** Daytime anxiety may also be helped by including CLA daily. You would need to take 1 softgel in the morning, again at noon and once more before 4 pm. Make sure to include 1 Ultimate Omega 3 in the morning and at noon along with one vitamin E in the morning.

We have tried to remove all trial and success out of this program but sometimes there are no other options. The Nature's Vitamin C, Probiotic Supreme and CLA daily are trial and success. They may not make a change or they may be the exact fit for your body. This is the stage to see if this is what your body needs to get over this hump.

If you have felt any improvement during these procedures, you have something to work with. If the anxiety has at least moved from a rating of 3 to a 5 and the anxiety is holding at that level using these supplements will be the answer for your success. You just need to adjust them further, allow a little additional time or adjust the time of day you are taking them. Adjust supplements one-by-one every third day. Keep good notes in your journal. The answers will either be the quantity taken of a supplement or it will be how often the supplement is taken. The answers will either be the quantity taken of a supplement or it will be how often the supplement is taken.

Experiment with this as needed and keep your Daily Journal. Give this some time to work. If you have had some improvement, such as from a 3 to a 5 rating and it is holding steady, but will not move beyond a 5 rating, give this stage 30 days to fully work.

After 30 days, if still at a 5 rating, move on to Step 2 and keep rating the daytime anxiety each evening. It may very well improve to a 7 rating later in the pre-taper.

You can have a blood test done and check the level of a substance called Interleukin-2 (IL-2). The reference range for IL-2 will be from 223 to 710 with most laboratories. If your test results come back with a level under 466, you need to increase the IL-2 further and you should increase the Beta 1, 3-D Glucan to 2500 me each day if needed. Increase by no more than 300 mg every 3 days.

If you have questions about the taper email:
info@theroadback.org
or call
866 892-0238
8:00 am – 3:30pm Tues-Thurs

ABOUT THE AUTHOR

Over the past thirty years, James Harper has owned successful businesses in the arena of telecommunications and financial services. His engineering viewpoint afforded him much success. But it was a conversation with his wife that brought awareness to the mass drugging of children in the American school system. Jim's disbelief in the drugging policies within education compelled him to search for the basic cause of symptoms that were misdiagnosed as psychiatric issues. However, the more he investigated the dais for the symptoms; it became apparent how prevalent the demand was for solutions. It was his background in engineering that provided the foundation for his research into drug withdrawals.

Jim spent many years researching the common denominators in withdrawal symptoms. He then applied the same research techniques to both the cause and treatment of these conditions that seemed to plague Mankind. The model he developed would set the stage for a powerful yet simple withdrawal program that could be applied mainstream. Through painstaking effort, the regimen in this book was perfected. Once he was assured the program was viable, Jim then responded to the mountain of request for assistance to taper off these medications.

In the past ten years, Jim has worked with countless individuals who wanted to taper off prescription medication and has trained medical doctors and psychiatrists in The Road Back Program for their practice. Jim's nutritional approach to tapering can gently taper an individual off psychoactive medication in weeks, instead of the normal months or even years. The Road back Program is now widely accepted by physicians worldwide who are using Jim's tapering method in their practice.

Made in the USA
Lexington, KY
30 April 2010